Praise for
Bee Miles

'An extraordinary twentieth century life. These pages dance with details of a forgotten Australia, in which the sane were in asylums, the rich were on the left and clever Bee Miles dominated the city of Sydney.'
Professor Alison Bashford, author of *An Intimate History of Evolution*

'The remarkable tale of an eternal vagabond, Bohemian to her core.'
Emeritus Professor Lucy Frost, historian and author

'A thrilling ride through the life of one of Australia's most gifted yet misunderstood characters. I adored it!'
Mandy Sayer, award-winning author

'Bee's defiant spirit leaps off every page in this brilliant rollercoaster of a book.'
Craig Munro, author of *Literary Lion Tamers*

Bee Miles

Bee Miles

Australia's famous bohemian rebel,
and the untold story behind the legend

Rose Ellis

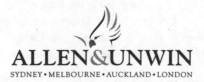

ALLEN&UNWIN

SYDNEY · MELBOURNE · AUCKLAND · LONDON

First published in 2023

Allen & Unwin
Cammeraygal Country
83 Alexander Street
Crows Nest NSW 2065
Australia
Phone: (61 2) 8425 0100
Email: info@allenandunwin.com
Web: www.allenandunwin.com

Allen & Unwin acknowledges the Traditional Owners of the Country on which we live and work. We pay our respects to all Aboriginal and Torres Strait Islander Elders, past and present.

A catalogue record for this book is available from the National Library of Australia

ISBN 978 1 76106 913 0

Index by Puddingburn Publishing Services
Set in 12/16 pt Adobe Garamond Pro by Midland Typesetters, Australia
Printed and bound in Australia by the Opus Group

10 9 8 7 6 5 4 3 2 1

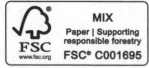

The paper in this book is FSC® certified. FSC® promotes environmentally responsible, socially beneficial and economically viable management of the world's forests.

For George and Betty with love and gratitude

'People are deathly afraid of both speaking and hearing the truth. And truth has been pictured as a naked woman. The average man fears her as he fears diseases, Lysol, fire, flood; and he comprehends her not at all.'

Bee Miles, 'I Leave in a Hurry'

Contents

Bee Miles

Preface

Bee Miles always maintained that she didn't want to be known, even though she lived most of her life under a public spotlight. A consummate performer and a perceptive critic, she was witness to each major change in Australia's fortunes during the last century: roaring prosperity, crippling financial depression and two world wars. In the 1920s she moved through its cities like 'the spirit of the age', personifying the confidence and defiance of youth and the optimism of a newly federated nation. In the 1930s she travelled across the country, overturning conventions that defined remote Australia as a male preserve. In the post-war 1940s and 1950s, when Sydney was subject to major reconstruction and women were being redirected back into the domestic sphere, she moved onto its streets and made them her home, where she worked, ate and slept under the public's gaze. It was a life punctuated by arrests, courtroom dramas, imprisonment and committals. By the time of her death in 1973 she had been arrested more than 300 times, had been in prisons and lockups in most parts of the country and had been a patient in at least seven psychiatric hospitals.

It is a strange thing to be famous for being homeless, yet Bee is perhaps best known for the way she lived in public places, as she moved her bedding between church doorways, parks and storm-water drains. For more than 50 years, she lived a very public life in towns and cities across the country—sleeping on their front steps, educating their sons and daughters, breaking their rules and living, as she liked to say, 'recklessly'. Through it all Bee remained circumspect about her own life, and about the circumstances that had taken her from the mansions of her childhood to the public parks and bandstands of her old age. And in that silence, the stories grew around her, stories that became legends, legends that became myths, and myths that became historical fact.

But all the while, the story of Bee's life, the key to many of the mysteries that so intrigued the public, was there. It travelled with her in a series of manuscripts that she wrote as she crossed and recrossed the country, as she sat in steaming outback police cells or in the brutal chaos of refractory wards or as she plied her trade on city streets as a roving reciter. Over her lifetime she completed five manuscripts that she tried unsuccessfully to have published. As narratives they are uneven, at times vivid, occasionally poignant, often humorous and always perceptive: Bee wrote from the margins, but she understood the centre. They are now housed in an archive in the NSW Mitchell Library and I have used them to guide me in the telling of Bee's story.

Bee always insisted that as a 'truth teller', she had to 'fly alone'. But the story of a life is comprised of multiple voices, including the relationships that help to define it. There are many people in this story whose lives intersected with Bee's, but no one had a greater influence than her father, William Miles. He is remembered in history as the founder of a hyper-nationalist independence movement in the 1930s, along with his editorial adviser 'Inky' Stephensen. But in the course of researching Bee's story, what has emerged is a far more complex figure, whose earlier commitment to the Left was as strong as his later alignment with the Right. His relationship with his daughter displayed the same contradictory elements. He raised her in a rationalist tradition that taught her to reject 'all forms of arbitrary authority' but when she began to question his own authority, their relationship fractured and led to him to becoming the principal actor in her committal as a psychiatric patient. As a result, she spent three years in the foetid hell of mental hospitals in her early twenties. She never forgave him for his betrayal, yet she was never able to let him go from her life either. Her time in the psychiatric hospitals honed the skills her father had taught her, and she learned to weaponise her resistance—something she would do for the rest of her life. She also left a record of her experiences that gives us a rare window into that world from the patient's perspective. That, as any researcher will tell you, is a priceless gift to history.

Other voices that emerge from this period and follow Bee through her life are contained in the hospital records over the period from the 1920s until the 1950s. They have been described as 'a palimpsest of early twentieth century Australian psychiatry'.[1] But they also reveal just how powerful and far-reaching notions of what was and was not acceptable behaviour for women were in controlling every aspect of their lives. And in Bee's case, just how devastating the consequences could be.

There is another figure in this story who remained unrecognised for many years. Bee never identified them or spoke of them, but they were there. This figure would come to affect almost aspect of her life, including her most important relationships. Her own silence about them in the pages of her manuscripts is matched by the silence of those charged with her care. Like the many other intriguing gaps in Bee's writing, it speaks volumes.

Terminology

Bee is referred to variously in this book as Bea, Bee and Beatrice. Apart from direct quotations, I have used the name Bee as that was always the way she preferred to be known. Some of the quotations in this book use language and terminology that are no longer acceptable to contemporary readers; however, in order to maintain historical accuracy, I have not attempted to alter the language within direct quotes.

1

On the Battlements

'The lack of unity among democrats is the only reason for autocracy's great power.'

William Miles, *The Socialist*, 22 March, 1918

The young girl sits at the piano at the end of the long room, under a huge bay window. From her seat she can see the sprawling gardens that surround the house and the fountain rising up from the circular driveway. A set of long stained-glass windows extend down from the vaulted ceiling. As the afternoon sun streams in from the west, it illuminates the figures who stare down at her as she plays. The faces of Haydn, Mozart and Beethoven surround her, watching sternly as she picks out the notes with her small fingers. Above the composers' heads stand the graceful figures of six women. Their faces are much gentler than the serious men at their feet. Some even seem playful. Each figure holds something different in her hands. One has a basket, another a scroll and another a musical instrument—the gifts of culture and industry.

The sun is starting to set now. As it recedes, fading beams fall upon another female figure watching the small girl. The woman is sitting straight-backed in a chair, dressed in a high-necked costume from another century. She has a strong face and a look that suggests she is not a woman to be trifled with. But there is kindness in her eyes and affection in her glance as she watches her granddaughter slowly and painfully sound out the notes on the grand piano. Now the room is almost dark, but the girl plays on, the sound of the piano echoing through the cavernous house. Everything else is silent. The girl, her grandmother and the music—nothing else. Just the way they like it.

———

Bee Miles was born on 17 September 1902 in the Sydney suburb of Summer Hill, the fourth of six children born to William John Miles and his wife Maria née Binnington. Her parents named her Beatrice, but she always preferred to be called Bee. For the first five years of her life she lived in Ashfield—a fast-developing suburb along the railway line, ten kilometres from the city—moving between her grandparents' and parents' residences. William Miles was the first member of his family to be born on Australian soil, and he and Bee would agitate for Australian independence throughout their lives.

William's grandfather, John Clement Miles, was the son of a Dover sea captain. John was a merchant who plied his trade between the colony of New South Wales and Tahiti, then a French protectorate known as the Society Isles. In 1843 he married Irish-born Martha Balfour, a farmer's daughter, at St James' Church in the centre of the newly declared city of Sydney, and returned with her to Tahiti, where he owned a restaurant and trading post. They lived there for several years before John died mysteriously and prematurely in a fire in the capital Papeete, at the age of 29. Martha, now a widow with two young children, returned to Australia in 1848, establishing her family in Woolloomooloo, then considered a rural retreat from the dusty streets of Sydney town.[1] Like many nineteenth-century widows, Martha Miles remarried. Her new husband was the colonial entrepreneur and inventor Allin Hollinshed, who like his new wife, owned several residences in and around Forbes Street.

6

Their combined holdings catered for a growing number of artisans and urban workers who had markedly increased Woolloomooloo's population over a decade, as one by one the fine mansions fell, and smaller rows of terrace houses grew in their place. Bee would later come to live in Woolloomooloo in the 1930s, though by then any hint of bucolic charm had disappeared.

John Balfour Clement Miles, Martha's son, grew up to be a successful accountant and investor. He established the accounting firm of Miles & Vane and became secretary of the Sydney Meat Preserving Company, where he was also a shareholder. This enterprise, which operated on 55 hectares (135 acres) at Haslam's Creek, (near what would later become Rookwood Cemetery), exported canned mutton to Britain and became a prosperous concern for the wealthy pastoralists who owned it. But John had another interest as well. He had purchased Peapes & Shaw, a popular clothing emporium in George Street. Both these investments would contribute to the family's growing wealth in the coming years.

Not far from Martha's Forbes Street terraces lay the small home of another Irish immigrant, William John Cordner, and his young English-born wife Ellen. Cordner was a leading musician and composer, and chief organist at St Mary's Cathedral. He is credited with modernising the cathedral's choir by opening it to the public and supporting female chorists, including his wife, who began as his student and quickly gained a reputation as the colony's finest contralto during the 1860s and 70s. The Cordners' small home in Cathedral Street became a centre for visiting musicians and performers. They were a talented couple who organised many successful public concerts and music festivals, including events associated with the opening of the Great Hall at Sydney University and the laying of the foundation stone at the Sydney Town Hall.[2] But they were artists rather than businesspeople, and although their works received positive reviews, they were often voluntary and they lived in penurious circumstances. When Cordner died in 1870, his friends and colleagues erected a large memorial at Rookwood

Cemetery to honour his contribution to both sacred and secular music.[3] The widowed Ellen moved into 174 Forbes Street, near the corner of what is now Cathedral Street, and became the tenant of Martha and Allin Hollinshed. Seven months later, at St Peter's Church, Woolloomooloo, she married John Balfour Clement Miles, the son of her landlady. She was already three months' pregnant with their first and only child, who was born on 27 August 1871. They named him William John—the same first two names as Ellen's former husband.

Ellen, who now performed under the name Mrs Cordner-Miles, continued to give public performances up to a month before her son was born, and was back performing four months later at the Prince of Wales Opera House.[4] This was highly unusual behaviour in a time when 'confinement' during pregnancy had a very literal meaning for middle-class women. The daughter of a Polish aristocrat, Ellen was described as having a 'regal presence' and a 'handsome figure' and was gifted with a 'ravishing' voice. She could sing both secular and sacred music with equal power, and when she performed, she was 'a whole contralto choir in herself'.[5] Her new husband was not an artist. His public performances were limited to interstate chess championships. But he was a savvy land speculator and in 1882 the family left Woolloomooloo, which by that stage had begun to acquire a reputation for overcrowding and violence, and set up residence in Ashfield, where William's father had purchased four-and-a-half hectares (eleven acres) of land.

The mansion Bee's grandfather built on Queen Street is still an imposing structure. Fortified by black iron gates, its Gothic Revival architecture dominates the surrounding bungalows that now occupy its former ample grounds. The music room, where a young Bee would learn the piano, remains one of its most outstanding features. Originally named Ambleside but known locally as Ashfield Castle, it was built in 1885 on two hectares (five acres) of land. On the remaining two-and-a-half hectares (six acres) he built three large houses, two of which remain: Kenilworth and Coniston, located in

Victoria Street just behind Ambleside. Coniston, where Bee lived with her parents, is an impressive Italianate gentleman's residence, originally designed with six bedrooms, stables and servants' quarters. Built five years before a crippling financial recession, these houses are expressions of opulence, optimism and grandeur; of European sensibilities and colonial ambition.

Unlike the somewhat precarious youth of his mother, William John Miles grew up in luxury. He was educated at the prestigious Newington School in Stanmore where he excelled in athletics. Like his father, he was a skilled chess player and became a state champion. Like his mother, he had a fine voice and sang regularly in St Mary's Cathedral choir and the Sydney Philharmonic Choir. His education was interrupted by frequent overseas travel with his parents. At the age of fourteen, he entered his father's accounting firm of Miles, Vane & Miles and embarked on what should have been a path devoted to commercial success and conservative values. In the former he succeeded. In the latter he diverged dramatically.[6]

The first divergence came when he crossed class lines to marry one of the household's servants, Maria Binnington, whose background was very different from her husband's. Maria's family had arrived in Brisbane in 1862 as bounty immigrants and were said to be distantly related to Sir Joseph Banks. The head of the family, Thomas Hodgson, was deeply religious and was shocked to learn that one of his daughters, Sarah, had fallen in love on the ship with a member of the crew, John Binnington. When the ship docked at Morton Bay, two-thirds of the crew deserted, including John. Sarah and John married at Ipswich in 1863 and had eight children. The seventh child was christened Maria, but was known by the family as 'Tot' because of her diminutive stature. During the 1890s depression, Maria relocated to Summer Hill in Sydney, where the extended Hodgson family had moved to improve their employment prospects. Maria gained a position at Ambleside as Ellen Miles' sewing maid and William fell in love with her.[7] William's mother did not attend the wedding of her only son,[8] and the newlyweds relocated to

Coniston, one of the mansions situated behind Ambleside. Within a few years the young family had moved to Wahroonga on Sydney's North Shore, where William had built an imposing home of his own on Cleveland Street. He named it after his hero, the naturalist Charles Darwin.

In 1908, when Bee was six years old, her grandfather died. He left a considerable estate worth around £42,000 that included majority shares in Peapes & Co., which had developed into a men's clothing store in George Street, opposite what would become Wynyard Station. William established himself as an independent consulting accountant with directorships of British General Electric and the Sydney Meat Preserving Company. He opened offices in Challis House in Martin Place opposite the GPO and only two blocks from the highly prosperous Peapes, where he now owned a 70 per cent share.

Details of Bee's childhood are scant. Her manuscripts and occasional published interviews do not dwell on her early years but focus on her late teens and early twenties and the domestic turbulence which dominated that period of her life. In an interview conducted shortly after Bee's death, Constance, her eldest sister, recalled that William was the central figure in the children's lives and that he was 'Victorian and strict'.[9] Although not a tall man, he had a presence that 'conveyed authority' and had a loud and rapid way of speaking.[10] The architect Hardy Wilson described him as 'an unusual man . . . so intelligent and without an instinct for beauty . . . he knew the importance of [it] and tried to understand'.[11] He also had a notoriously ferocious temper.[12] At the same time, William appears to have been an indulgent parent, often showering his offspring with gifts and dressing up as Father Christmas every year, even when the children were older. In many ways it was an idyllic life. There were bush picnics, tennis parties and outings to concerts or the opera. There were holidays to the Central Coast and Palm Beach, where William eventually bought a holiday home on Sunrise Road, christening it Darwinia, after the native flower.[13] There the family took their leisure with other wealthy families who owned holiday homes or rented them for the Christmas holiday period, where their activities were reported regularly in the social pages.

Music was an important part of family life. Although she didn't inherit her grandmother's fine singing voice, Bee excelled as a pianist. The family often sang around the piano while she played. In a rare childhood memory, she recalled evenings when: 'My sisters and brothers and I would tap on the table the rhythm of various songs and pieces of music—bits from Grand Opera, from Beethoven, Mozart, Chopin and jazz—and would sneer frightfully at any of us that couldn't recognise the tune intended.'[14]

William had an extensive library, which included works by T.H. Huxley, Herbert Spencer and Charles Darwin. Bee was an avid reader from an early age, which her father encouraged. She had an obvious facility for memorising and reciting poetry, and the works of Shakespeare were a central part of her repertoire. William was a member and honorary treasurer of the New South Wales Shakespeare Society, which Professor Mungo MacCallum, Dean of Arts at Sydney University, had established in 1902. Together with his wife Maria, William took part in the Society's annual performances, including an event in 1912 that was held to raise funds for the Shakespeare monument, which now sits opposite the Mitchell Library. The Society was also instrumental in the creation of the Shakespeare Room within the library itself: the same library on whose steps Bee would ply her trade as reciter of Shakespeare decades later and which would eventually ban her for smoking.

Bee and her sisters, Constance and Louise, attended Abbotsleigh College in Wahroonga, while her brothers, John and Arthur, were educated at Sydney Grammar. Helen, their parents' first child, had died as an infant. William admired his daughter Bee's intelligence and was pleased with the way she impressed adults from an early age with her extensive general knowledge. She was more fortunate than her siblings. William would frequently quiz them on a range of subjects and castigate them so severely when they gave the wrong answers that their mother had to comfort them. A proponent of free thought and rationalism, he raised his children as atheists. They were not allowed to attend church or Sunday school or allowed to have any religious training at school. When Constance returned home one day complaining that her teacher had claimed that evolutionary theory was spurious, William went down to Abbotsleigh and 'raised Cain'.[15]

While he was a successful accountant and merchant, William's passions and politics took him in a very different direction from the commercial world and the upper-middle-class life he had built for his family. Two seminal events in his youth started him on a path that would not only frame the philosophical outlook of his daughter, but also drag his family's reputation into controversy. The first was witnessing the colonies win the Ashes against England in 1882, which he later claimed instilled in him a strong sense of nationalism and made him a 'convinced Australian'. The second was watching New South Wales troops pass through the Woolloomooloo Gates on their way to Sudan to fight under the British flag three years later, when he was fourteen years of age. The sight of Australians leaving to fight in a battle so far removed from their own soil created a sense of injustice that would never leave him.[16]

William had come to adulthood in the fading days of the Australian republican movement, but he was more than ready for the turbulent politics that replaced it. The free thought and rationalist movement he came to embrace gained currency in the mid to late nineteenth century, following the publication of Darwin's *The Origin of Species*. The Rationalist Press was founded in London in 1885 and was the leading publisher of free thought and secular literature. It defined rationalism as: 'The mental attitude which accepted the primacy of reason with the aim to establish a system of philosophy and ethics verifiable by experience and independent of all arbitrary assumptions or authority.'[17]

Years later Bee would write her own definition of rationalism in a song she composed for atheist children:

I'm an Atheist born and bred
I don't come alive once I'm dead
I'm sound in the body and sane in the head
I'm an Atheist born and bred.
I'm an Atheist by conviction
The Bible, I think, is mostly fiction
Idiotic stories but magnificent diction
I'm an Atheist by conviction.
I'm an Atheist because I've thought
I try to be good because I ought
And not because I think I'll go to hell if I'm caught
I'm an Atheist because I've thought.[18]

Proving her atheism was relatively easy. Proving she was 'sane in the head' was something Bee would find increasingly difficult throughout her adult life.

William Miles became the representative of the Rationalist Press in Australia and organised lecture tours for international freethought advocates, including the controversial former priest turned rationalist, Joseph McCabe. In 1912 he established the New South Wales Rationalist Association, which attracted more members than any other state branch.[19] He published a pamphlet entitled *The Myth of the Resurrection of Jesus Christ* and issued public challenges to senior church leaders to debate the validity of religion. Many socialist groups were aligned with or were generated by the freethought movement, and William began to develop associations that would have filled his corporate colleagues with both puzzlement and disdain.

———

The year 1916 was a pivotal one. Fissures began to erupt across the political landscape, and within the Miles family, the facade of a genteel upper-middle-class domestic life began to shatter. Recalling that difficult time, still fresh in her memory after fifty years, Bee observed:

> He [William] loved me till I was about fourteen. After that he started to hate me . . . because he was frightfully jealous, not only of me but of Grandma and of all the children before I was fourteen. He resented Grandma because she had all the money and he had to go to her for it [and] . . . because we were going to inherit that money.[20]

Adolescence is a difficult time in many families. Nascent independence, often cloaked in minor acts of rebellion, starts to emerge. In the Miles family it was made more complicated by the fact that William had encouraged his children to be independent thinkers from an early age and follow the rationalist dictum to reject all forms of 'arbitrary assumptions or authority'. No doubt he didn't consider his own authority as arbitrary. Perhaps aware of his limited formal education, which had been constantly interrupted by overseas travel with his parents, there appeared to be some intellectual rivalry between William and his daughter. While proud of her burgeoning intellect, Bee would later state that her father was jealous of it as well: 'Because I was more intelligent, better educated, had a great deal more intellectual and moral courage, an infinitely better memory and superior by birth . . . He's ten per cent Bilenski, I'm 99 per cent.'[21]

William's grandfather, Count Ferdinand Bilenski—a Polish aristocrat, writer and political agitator—was one of the few relatives both Bee and her father ever discussed publicly. Though neither of them had ever met him, they both liked to boast about how much they resembled him. Bilenski, who'd been exiled to Siberia before escaping to France, had met and married Ellen's mother in Paris. Like her son (and possibly her father, the count), Ellen was a formidable woman who liked to dress in the style of the French Empress Eugenie.[22] It is not hard to imagine a clash of wills between mother and son, particularly if she had control of the considerable estate left by her husband. But she also loved her talented granddaughter, and it was Ellen who eventually gave Bee a small allowance to provide her with some independence from her father a few years later, when their relationship was particularly fraught. When things at home became difficult, as they frequently did, Bee sought refuge with her grandmother, who was then living in Strathfield.

Family friction is a battle fought daily. Superficial wounds heal quickly in readiness for the next inevitable confrontation. But parental rejection leaves scars that are deep and enduring. The sense of betrayal that Bee must have felt as her once-indulgent father began to replace his affection with animosity would build over the following years to become unbearable. Looking back at that period, she would later claim that if she had to live her life again from the age of fourteen to twenty-five, 'I'd commit suicide'.[23] For the rest of her life, she saw herself as utterly 'unlovable'.

Political tensions outside the home were growing too. The First World War was in its third year and initial support for Australian involvement began to wane as casualty numbers rose. Despite British demands for 5500 troops a month, enlistment numbers started to decline. When jingoistic recruitment campaigns exploiting Australia's British loyalties failed to meet the increasing need for more recruits, Labor Prime Minister Billy Hughes mooted the idea of compulsory enlistment through conscription.

The Anti-Conscription League of New South Wales had already been established in 1915, predominantly by the Industrial Workers of the World (IWW), a movement whose espousal of direct action rather than arbitration filled industrialists, employer groups and governments with alarm.[24] Their leader, Tom Barker, had been arrested on sedition charges but was released after a strident political campaign.[25] The league met weekly over the course of nearly two years and drew together socialists, feminists, pacifists, politicians and militants. It also attracted William John Miles, who represented the Rationalist Association. He soon became a regular speaker at the

Domain, addressing huge crowds drawn to the Sunday meetings, both for their political messages and their entertainment value. It would have been an odd spectacle: the wealthy merchant and avowed atheist sharing the stage with the Reverend Albert Rivett and militant IWW members. He was, from all reports, an effective speaker, and in an age without microphones he held the audience's attention with his 'precise, rapid and loud voice'.[26] Like his mother and his daughter, William had a penchant for performance.

The Domain had, at least from the turn of the century, offered a dedicated forum for free speech. On Sunday afternoons it was a common sight to see crowds moving from speaker to speaker, each atop makeshift platforms, all vying for their attention, hoping for a donation and perhaps even a conversion. During the First World War, the mood was different. Walking down Oxford Street on a Sunday afternoon, a young Lewis Rodd, future husband of the novelist Kylie Tennant, described the crowds heading for the Domain as:

> an army on the march, an army of men and women bitter, disillusioned, most of them elderly whose political idols, the Holmans and the Hugheses, had proved to have feet of brass . . . At the corner of Hyde Park where the new Wentworth Avenue joined with College Street came another steadily marching almost silent group from Ultimo, Glebe and Redfern . . . and at the Domain gates joined with two more, one surging up from Woolloomooloo and the other coming across the city from the Rocks.[27]

These were dangerous days. Fiery speeches attracted spectators, but they also drew the attention of the police, moving through the crowds in plain clothes and taking notes on any comments that could be viewed as disloyal or seditious. Twelve IWW members were arrested and found guilty of conspiracy to commit sedition and arson after a series of fires around the city in 1916.[28] Many of the Left saw this as an attempt to shut down the anti-conscription campaigns. In fact, it had the opposite effect. The imprisonment of the twelve galvanised the Left; campaigns for their release were led by prominent journalists and Labor parliamentarians. It was a volatile world and William thrived in it.

Away from the speaker's box, William funded the production of pamphlets arguing that 'no Australian should be forcibly transported to Europe and made to fight there against his will'.[29] These and other campaign materials were subsequently banned. He also worked closely with Melbourne Archbishop Daniel Mannix, who galvanised the Catholic vote in opposition to conscription. Despite his often-militant stance towards organised religion, William would have had many contacts within the hierarchy of the Catholic Church, where his mother was still extremely well regarded. The campaign was bitter and those opposed to conscription were accused of both cowardice and disloyalty to the Empire. Feminists campaigning against the war were physically attacked, including Adela Pankhurst Walsh, who, together with her husband Tom, was also a member of the Anti-Conscription League, and a future foundation member of the Communist Party.[30] While Prime Minister Hughes appealed to women to send their sons to war as 'the proud mothers of a nation of heroes' or risk being 'dishonoured as the mothers of a race of degenerates',[31] feminists like Rose Scott, who had led the campaign for female suffrage, joined forces with the Quakers to argue against the barbarity and violence of war.

At Bee's school, patriotic support for the war and loyalty to Britain were inextricably linked and equally fervent. Bee and her sisters were instructed by their father to wear 'No' badges to school during two referenda campaigns. This caused considerable controversy and placed the girls in the spotlight as the only dissenters in the school.[32] Many students and teachers had lost relatives during the war, including neighbouring families in Bee's street. With the word 'No' conspicuously pinned to the front of her uniform, Bee was often forced to defend her father in clashes with both her classmates and her teachers, and while her sisters disliked the attention, she relished the controversy and opportunity for debate. It was not reciprocated by her teachers; although her early years at Abbotsleigh appear to have been relatively happy, things began to change dramatically.

Bee described her teachers as 'rabid jingoist[s]', one of whom indulged in 'bitter invective against the Germans' during class, describing them as 'Huns'. Things came to a head when Bee was given an English composition assignment on 'The True Significance of the Gallipoli Campaign':

> Of course I asked at home and was told by my father, who had remained quite sane all through the war years, that its true significance was that it was a strategical blunder. That was the tenor of my essay. The rest of the girls, harking to the chauvinist, wrote essays to the effect that it was a wonderful effort. I got low marks and they were praised.[33]

Employing the rationalist framework in which she had been raised, Bee began to reject what she increasingly saw as the 'arbitrary authority' of her teachers and the discipline of the school. Looking back on that period, two decades on, her resentment over her treatment was still strong:

> With a few exceptions I have nothing now but contempt for my mistresses and companions. How many times the principal threatened to expel me I can't recall. It was for nothing more than riotousness and disobedience. If I had been a cheat, a liar or thief there would have been excuse for expulsion but what child of reasonable personality isn't riotous and disobedient with women, especially with mistresses of private schools or any other sort of school?[34]

The word 'frivolous' began to appear more frequently in Bee's school reports.[35]

Outside the domestic sphere, William's activities were also drawing controversy. He established two organisations, the No Imperial Federation League and the Advance Australia League.[36] His successes as a Domain speaker led him to embark on inter-state tours, with his speeches praised in the socialist press.[37] The conscription battles of 1916–17 were largely drawn along class lines, which placed the commercially successful William in a curious position. Middle- and upper-class populations generally supported conscription, while the anti-conscription campaigns were spearheaded by unionists and socialists, who also supported the campaign to free the imprisoned IWW members. Anti-industrialist and anti–war profiteering sentiment was strong amongst these groups, who saw the European conflict as a 'capitalists' war'. As a successful business owner and a member of the Chamber of Commerce, William was one of those capitalists. But, unlike his contemporaries, he moved in both professional and radical circles simultaneously. Although he was always careful in business invest-ment, there was a recklessness about him. He would travel from his well-appointed offices in Challis House down to the Trades Hall in Sussex Street to speak at meetings, willing to risk his professional reputation and potentially his clientele if he believed sufficiently in a cause. Having to pass the recruitment centre that had been set up so prominently at the GPO opposite his office in Martin Place on his way would only have increased both his chagrin and his commitment. At a time when anti-German senti-ment was at fever pitch, he attempted to visit rationalists who had been interned because of their German heritage; at Challis House, surrounded by the nation's wealthiest insurance companies and banks, he openly entertained veteran IWW radicals in his offices.[38] Even his cultural pursuits became controversial. In 1916 he was asked to resign from the New South Wales Shakespeare Society, due to 'his constant opposition' at meetings. Professor MacCallum and many of the members were ardent supporters of the Empire and conscription. William refused to resign.[39]

Eventually, despite two referenda, the conscription campaign was defeated, and Hughes along with other pro-conscriptionists left the Labor Party and formed the Nationalist Party. Opposition to the war and to the imprisonment of IWW members continued and there were multiple arrests for sedition under the *War Precautions Act* amongst Domain speakers. William appeared as a witness for the defence in two notable trials that attracted widespread media attention.[40] Shortly afterwards his home was raided and printed materials seized, particularly those relating to the Advance Australia League.[41]

2

Trouble on the
North Shore Line

'There's a glamour of a diabolic, miserable sort attached to wandering, unhappy, uneasy unkind rebel sons; but what about daughters—daughters who will not conform have no glamour, respect or love: what they have in mind interests no-one. They have no position in society—and what man will ever marry them?'

Christina Stead, 'The Solitaries, the Submitted, the Wanderers'

By the early twentieth century, Wahroonga, an upper North Shore suburb of Sydney, had become an area for affluent professionals to build impressive homes, many of which are now heritage listed because of their architectural significance. Most households had live-in domestic staff and tradesmen entered the properties through the rear. Children were educated at the various prestigious private schools that dotted the area, and generations of families moved in select and insular social circles. Politics were conservative and class lines were tightly drawn. Prominent families included members of the Anthony Horden dynasty and the artist Lionel Lindsay, who presented Bee's sister Constance with a painting as a wedding gift. A police raid and the taint of political scandal in this wealthy and secluded suburb must have caused some embarrassment for the Miles family, but it did not deter William. During 1918 he remained active in radical circles and wrote regularly for socialist publications, while continuing his role as secretary of the New South Wales Rationalist Association. Bee was in her senior year at Abbotsleigh and, despite her clashes with the principal, she was one of thirteen classmates who passed their leaving exams, gaining an Honours in English and B passes in Latin, French and History.

At home the tensions that had been building steadily since she was fourteen had turned into open battle. Bee's refusal to submit to discipline led to extreme and 'stormy scenes' regarding her 'wilful behaviour'. Bee rarely spoke about her mother, though she had enjoyed a close relationship with her as a child, which she later described as a 'fixation'. This changed when she turned sixteen and the fights between them became particularly hostile.[1] Bee later observed that her mother grew jealous of her close relationship with her father. 'If he danced at all, he danced with me, he didn't dance with her,' she said, adding that her mother was justified to resent the attention her daughter was receiving.[2] But according to William, Bee had developed a 'fixation' on him 'owing to her particular hostility to her mother'. It was clear to him 'that some special jealousy was operating with Beatrice, and in a scene with her I told her that if she was trying to alienate her mother and me from one another she was attempting the impossible and merely "running her head against a stone wall"'.[3]

Shifting allegiances, familial jealousies and passionate quarrels became an almost daily occurrence. A particular source of tension was Bee's interest in 'sex knowledge'. It was a topic that her parents found difficult to discuss—despite William's championing of evolutionary theory and rational debate. Perhaps he resented Bee's precociousness and perceived this constant questioning as a challenge to his intellect and his parental authority. This was an era where sex education in schools was non-existent and access to publications that discussed sexuality or advertised contraceptives was legally restricted.

Church groups and sections of the medical profession strongly supported prohibitions on publications discussing sexuality or advertising contraceptives, though they could be found in the rationalist and free thought bookshops promoted by Bee's father through the Rationalist Association.[4] Young, single women, despite their increased mobility and education, were still expected to apply restraint and remain virginal until married.[5] The information Bee was seeking was out of bounds for a schoolgirl, and the answers that her parents supplied were deemed at best unsatisfactory and at worst dishonest. The role of sexuality in human society was a topic that would continue to preoccupy Bee in her writing for most of her life. Like the writer Christina Stead (whose father was also an atheist and a rationalist), who wrote so descriptively of the sexual yearning of her youth, Bee maintained a lifelong belief that sexual repression led to 'madness'.[6]

In early 1920 Bee was preparing to sit her entrance examinations for Sydney University when she became seriously ill. In the many newspaper reports and vignettes about Bee over the years, her 'eccentric' behaviour was often ascribed to a nervous breakdown caused by 'over study' in her first year of university. As the veteran journalist and author Gavin Souter once observed, 'over-study rarely turns the mind'.[7] In fact, Bee had contracted encephalitis lethargica, a disease that had emerged in Europe during the First World War and became a pandemic.

Encephalitis lethargica was a seriously debilitating disease with a high mortality rate. During the early twentieth century it swept through Europe and Australia causing 500,000 deaths.[8] Young people were particularly susceptible. Bee's symptoms first became noticeable when buying gloves with her mother at Farmer's department store. She fell asleep at the counter and the staff were unable to wake her.[9] The symptoms continued when she was taking a maths exam. Her vision deteriorated and she 'felt she was going to die'.[10] There were, in fact, questions about her survival. The doctor informed her family that her condition would either be fatal or leave her with serious side effects.[11]

While many people did survive the disease and recovered, most had severe and lifelong symptoms that varied between Parkinsonism, photosensitivity, obesity, prolonged sleep states, hyperkinetic behaviour, exhibitionism and distractedness.[12] Some symptoms appeared immediately, while others developed over time. Because the disease primarily affected younger people, many survivors suffered the side effects for decades afterwards. The book *Awakenings*, by neurologist Oliver Sacks, explores the impact of encephalitis lethargica on a group of catatonic patients, some forty years after they were first infected. While Bee, even in her later years, did not display any signs of Parkinsonism, such as tremors, stiffness or slowed movements, she did wear an eyeshade—possibly due to her sensitivity to light—and she also started to become obese in her early forties. But, for the rest of her life, Bee was addicted to movement and to risk. (It's hard to read Marinetti's *Manifesto of Futurism* without thinking of her.) She loved to move fast, and she loved the machines that moved her. She began with trains, charging on when they were departing and jumping off just before they stopped, then progressed to trams and ferries before perfecting her skills with moving cars—though this was slightly later.

Despite the debilitating nature of her illness, Bee successfully passed the entrance examinations for Sydney University. She had considered a career in medicine, and qualified for entry into the schools of Medicine, Science and Law, but she eventually chose Arts, majoring in Philosophy and English. Before she commenced her studies, her father had taken her to see the prominent psychiatrist Dr Chisholm Ross—who would become a notorious figure for Bee in a few years' time. William had consulted him to see if his daughter 'could, without danger to herself, proceed to the University'.[13] She must have been pronounced capable of study because in 1921 she joined a small but growing group of female undergraduates.

Bee attended university every day, travelling by steam train from Wahroonga to Milsons Point, then by ferry across the harbour and then a tram to Sydney University. To her father's intense annoyance and no doubt to the family's mortification, her behaviour started to attract attention and she began to be known as 'mad Bee Miles' on the North Shore Line because of her constant jumping on and off moving trains. She had also started to leap onto trams, and thus began the first of five decades of court appearances when she appeared at Glebe Court and was fined for boarding a moving tram.[14] Within the highly conservative and male-oriented environment of the university, Bee was also drawing attention. She often chose to attend lectures in tennis attire, occasionally accompanied by a dog and increasingly late each time. When she appeared, the male students would stamp their feet until the lecturer finally had to ask them to desist, claiming the young woman 'was not quite right'. The next time Bee attended a lecture she was greeted by silence. She never returned.[15]

Having completed only one year of undergraduate study, she then enrolled at the Kindergarten Training College in Darlinghurst but only lasted a couple of months. According to her father this was due to complaints from the other students. Bee later claimed it was because she hated children.[16] In 1922 she went to stay at a holiday home near Goulburn. Either the family sent her there to gain some respite, or she took herself. She had planned to stay several weeks but the trip was cut short after a few days. Her father claimed that she attacked the proprietor's daughter, hitting her 'or catching her by the throat'. She was examined by Dr Roger Cope who, according to her father, thought she should be placed in an asylum.[17]

Following this incident William put his daughter in the care of Dr B.M. Carruthers, initially for 'disciplinary and . . . psychoanalytic treatment', although he later acknowledged it was actually 'to get final proof, as far as possible . . . that Beatrice's trouble was a psychosis as distinct from a neurosis'.[18] Bee later claimed that it was her father's first serious attempt to have her 'put away'. During her treatment she stayed with a nurse, Miss Symes, in Ashfield and the psychiatrist visited her daily. After six weeks Dr Carruthers voluntarily relinquished his patient, claiming that her 'trouble was only neurotic'.[19]

In the following year Bee enrolled in a shorthand and typing course at Scott & Underwood in George Street, where her apparent failure to follow instruction again resulted in complaints by teachers and fellow students. She did manage to complete the course, although she later conceded that she could never get the speed required for shorthand. There was a brief attempt at independent living when Bee moved into a boarding house in North Sydney for a few weeks in October 1923. She soon incurred the wrath of her landlady by playing the piano at four in the morning. Her piece of choice was Chopin's 'Funeral March'. She was threatened with eviction and returned to Wahroonga.[20]

Back at home the volatility and the violence escalated. Both parents, and by now the siblings, were exasperated by Bee's behaviour and, she claimed, were urged on by their father to retaliate with violence: 'He'd say to my brothers and sisters and mother "be nasty to her ... hit her, hit her" and so help me, goodness those poor things that they were, they did. Not because they were nasty and violent. They were neither. But because they were so dominated by my father.'[21]

The violence, recalled in such detail fifty years later, seemed to erupt over the most mundane domestic disputes, particularly between Bee and her father. Years later, when pressed by an interviewer about why her father was so cruel, she remarked, 'The only case I can think about like my father's was Barrett of Wimpole Street, but he loved his daughter ... my father hated me.'[22] It was as if her very presence in the family home infuriated him:

> He'd mock me about the most trivial things ... if I gave
> him a cup and the handle wasn't turned directly towards
> him, he'd jump up and slap my face. If I sighed or frowned

or looked out the window . . . he'd rush at me and start knocking me about, slapped my face and punched me. One day I had the crumb tray on the table . . . to pick up the crumbs. He said, 'What are you doing with that?' I said, 'So the crumbs won't fall on the floor'. He said, 'Don't argue,' and knocked me down. But I hadn't argued. I had only answered his question.[23]

In a series of letters to Bee's doctors, William claimed that many of their disputes centred around his daughter's refusal to do her share of domestic work, her untidiness and her choice of wardrobe. William thought that the way his daughter dressed—as lightly as possible—'evidenced her insanity as clearly as anything'.[24] Her failure to keep her bedroom tidy seemed to be a particular source of irritation for her parents. Clothing was strewn about the room, along with 'books, music and knick-nacks [sic]'. She had also developed a habit of taking extremely long hot baths, followed by cold showers. The time she spent in the bathroom was so long, her father claimed, that they had to install an extra bath in another room for the rest of the family. She became critical of the meals that were cooked for her and demanded 'fancy foods'. Food became such an issue that it had to be 'locked up to stop her picking'. He also acknowledged that he had to use 'force' with her—'I have sometimes had to hit her severely'—but that he suspected that she had provoked it, 'for the sake of being hit'. The beatings used to leave him 'frazzled for half an hour afterwards'.[25] Bee, he added, was violent as well, often striking her mother and sister, along with their housekeeper during disputes over housework.[26] When his daughter was present, he wrote, 'normal homelife was absent'.[27]

The minute detail with which William described each facet of his daughter's behaviour as a symptom of her 'insanity' is curious. It reads like a catalogue of dysfunction, created and submitted as evidence. And perhaps that's what it was—the rationalist attempting to compile 'verifiable' facts. But it also reads like the outpourings of someone whose daily life had become an intolerable nightmare, where the simplest domestic routines had become exhausting, unwinnable battles. According to Bee, her father had been taking notes on her misdemeanours for several years: 'When I was 18, he hated me so much that he wanted me locked up . . . he tried to drive me mad. He'd go around with a piece of paper and pencil and write down in a book everything that he thought about me was mad. Such a person is insane himself.'[28]

———

William's political activities were also coming under increasing strain. He had continued his speaking tours and his contributions to leftist publications like *The Australian Worker*, *The Socialist*, *Ross's Monthly* and the free thought journal *The Liberator*. He worked with Bertha McNamara—prominent socialist and feminist, proprietor of the Free Thought Bookshop and mother-in-law to both Jack Lang and Henry Lawson—to raise funds for the dependants of the still-incarcerated IWW men. In what William acknowledged was a final and futile act, he tried to unite several socialist groups to form a coalition and his failure led him to despair.[29] In 1920 he terminated his association with the New South Wales Rationalist Association, claiming they were agnostic rather than truly atheistic and far too focused on the middle class.[30]

Despite his overt socialist leanings, the mixed fortunes of his political forays and his railing against the 'greed of the wealthy classes',[31] William's own business enterprises continued to thrive. Peapes & Co. was well established as a leading men's wear store, ranking in prestige and reputation with David Jones, Anthony Horden's and Farmer's as a major retail outlet and men's outfitter of distinction. The majority of Sydney's private school boys were outfitted at Peapes, and clever marketing and fine workmanship had made a handmade shirt or a golfing outfit from Peapes' famous Warrigal range a status symbol for their older brothers and fathers.

The store offered a meeting place or informal club for customers visiting the city, while its sales representatives travelled across the country, where they hired rooms in hotels so that rural customers and their male offspring could travel in for fittings. Peapes' logo was 'for men and their sons'. In 1923 the store underwent a refurbishment on a grand scale. Its new building opposite Hunter Street at 285 George Street, with its Georgian facade and rich Queensland maple interiors, was seen as an elegant antidote to the pedestrian nature of other contemporary developments, in a city that was undergoing significant change. Elliptical wells reached down through its seven floors extending natural light to the centre from its rooftop dome. It was designed by Hardy Wilson, an esoteric and idiosyncratic architect who became increasingly antisemitic in the interwar period and would be drawn into future controversy through his continued association with William. The new building had a grand opening on 17 December, attracting the city's leading merchants as well as Sydney Ure Smith, president of the Society of Artists and, somewhat ironically, the archbishop. The New South Wales Premier George Fuller officially opened the building and, in a rather pointed speech, described Peapes as evidence of the progress that could be achieved when labour, government and industry worked in harmony. He also warned against socialist forces that sought to undermine and disrupt the current government's agenda.[32]

William, although the major shareholder and director, was absent from the opening. In fact, he was largely absent from all public life. He would re-emerge a decade later, stripped of his socialist and democratic loyalties and plunge his family and associates into a political maelstrom from which none would survive unscathed. But in December 1923, after spending so much energy and money on the politics of his passions, he disappeared from public view. Historians have assumed that he used this period to concentrate on growing his business interests, but the reason may have been much closer to home.

At the beginning of December, weeks away from the grand opening of the new Peapes store, the violence in the house had reached a crescendo. Amid all the turbulence, the way in which Maria Miles responded to her daughter is unclear. In many ways she remains the off-stage presence behind this unrelenting domestic drama. Bee once said that she was 'too quiet' and didn't like her bringing friends to the house.[33] William had always claimed that they were a united front in opposition to their daughter's behaviour. But on this night, she stepped into the spotlight and placed herself firmly between her husband and her daughter. William had beaten Bee so badly that Maria threatened to go to the police. Instead, William took his daughter to the Lunatic Reception House at Darlinghurst.[34] It was three weeks before Christmas and Bee was twenty-one years of age. She was 5 foot 5 inches tall (1.65 metres) with bobbed brown hair and clear blue eyes. She was slim, educated, eloquent and attractive. As the *Police Gazette* arrest notices later noted, with no apparent sense of irony, she was 'good looking and appears intelligent'.[35]

3

Wanting in Control

'It takes a man or woman of great moral courage—a man or woman almost unique—to dare the risk of being himself or herself all the time, never posing, acting or affecting. It is a dangerous business being yourself. I know of nothing more certain to provoke the almost always false epithet 'mad' or to deprive that man or woman of his or her liberty.'

Bee Miles, 'Dictionary by a Bitch', p. 1

The early twentieth century's obsession with progress, efficiency and racial destiny saw the development of a number of ways to classify, separate and at times isolate different sections of society, which varied according to race, class and gender.[1] In newly federated Australia, for example, the precarious nature of whiteness and the fear of racial degeneracy preoccupied legal, medical and political debate, which in turn influenced legislation.[2] One of the most pernicious examples was the forced removal of Indigenous children from their families, particularly in the interwar period. This practice utilised the category of race to classify, separate and isolate children and adults into different institutions in order to 'absorb' mixed race offspring into the broader white community, while controlling the movement of their parents. Similarly, ideas about moral and physical contamination influenced the way that individuals with perceived mental disorders were classified and treated within the medical and welfare systems, by using the categories of 'fit' and 'unfit'. Within the category of the unfit, subcategories of curable and incurable were formed, allowing greater official intervention into the private lives of citizens than in any other preceding period.[3]

In the first half of the twentieth century these aspects of eugenic theory remained ubiquitous and influential. Fear of the broader population's physical and moral contamination led to the formation of various social reform movements, including racial and mental hygienists. They attracted an eclectic membership of educators, politicians, moral reformers, feminists and doctors from both the Right and Left of politics. Their concerns were twofold: the spread of venereal disease, particularly after the First World War; and the perceived rise in 'feeble-minded' people in the community. Over the decades concerns about the contaminating properties of feeble-mindedness were broadened to include the 'mentally and socially inefficient'. This category included prostitutes, homosexuals, the poor and criminals.[4] Psychiatrists were strong proponents of the notion of inherited defects and the apparent need to separate the feeble-minded and the unfit from wider society, and argued for increased control over what they saw as problem populations, including the category of 'feeble-minded women'.[5] The lunatic, who in previous generations had required protection from society, had now become defective and was potentially harmful to future generations.[6]

There was a common belief that the 'insane' had less ability to apply sexual restraint and, because their 'defects' were hereditary, this made 'feeble-minded' women particularly dangerous. The 1912 *Maternity Allowance Act*, for example, came under considerable attack by the Charity Organisation Society because of its universal application to all (white) women, regardless of marital status. This was seen as encouraging the proliferation of moral degenerates and disrupting the organisation's process of characterising recipients into 'deserving' or 'undeserving' of charity.[7] During the first decades of the twentieth century, several politicians, physicians and social reformers advocated involuntary sterilisation of the unfit,[8] as the language of moral, social and political reform became increasingly medicalised. Bad seed had entered the social body.

Unlike other countries, including the United States, Canada and parts of Europe, sterilisation laws were never passed in Australia.[9] But it did share similar concerns about 'unfit' females and their capacity to reproduce defective children, which was mirrored in committal patterns. During the 1920s men were more highly represented in initial admissions to psychiatric care, but women were more likely to be readmitted after release. Between 1880 and 1930, 40 per cent of all psychiatric patients were single women. Up until 1914 these patients were largely prostitutes, recalcitrant domestic servants and vagrants, but in subsequent years they were replaced by single, urban women either living in boarding houses or with their parents.[10] Women like Bee Miles.

———

It must have been a long and difficult journey on that summer's day on the second of December 1923, when William took his daughter from their comfortable home in Wahroonga to the Reception House in Forbes Street, Darlinghurst. The location of this imposing Victorian building, adjacent to Darlinghurst Gaol, was deliberate. Opened in 1868, the Reception House held prisoners who were arrested on suspicion of insanity under temporary detention until they were clinically examined, and the nature of their disturbance determined. In addition, the introduction of the Reception House enabled patients who might not prove certifiable, or whose behaviour might be a temporary lapse—for example alcohol-related—to avoid the stigma of being sent to an asylum. It was also the place where private citizens could bring family members for committal.

Following the legal requirements of the period, Bee was examined by two psychiatrists, Dr Gibbes and Dr Chisholm Ross—the same psychiatrist who had assessed her as suitable for university study two years before. Even now there was little in the two doctors' observations to substantiate a committal under the *Lunacy Act* and no mention of her recent illness, although it did appear in her later case notes.[11] Instead, the report focused on her intractable behaviour:

> That she cannot get on with her home folks and never can; that she does not work domestically, that she does travel on trains without money and is often away from home without reason. She is childish and markedly wanting in control. Very excited, talks rapidly and constantly, confesses that she is in the habit of boarding moving vehicles and riding in public conveyances without paying her fare ... Statement by father indicates she has been eccentric and uncontrollable at home and acts irresponsibly in public. [Bee] would like to become a movie actress.[12]

Closer analysis of these comments reveals more about the observers than the object of their gaze. In the early twentieth century, gendered perceptions about what constituted acceptable female behaviour appeared consistently in judicial and medical discourse and this had serious implications for the constraint of women. A loss of interest in or a refusal to carry out domestic duties was often seen as a justification for committal.[13]

Bee Miles, though neither poor nor feeble-minded, but seemingly 'socially inefficient' and lacking in control, fell into this category when she was brought to the Reception House for psychiatric assessment. There would be a stage in the future when Bee came to embrace aspects of eugenic theory for her own brand of nationalism, but, at this moment in time, surrounded by two government-appointed psychiatrists and her own well-connected father, she was its casualty.

When Bee reflected on the experience afterwards, her own version of what led her there was very different from her father's overly detailed explanations:

> Dad appears to be eliminating me from the family. He tried to have me put away a year or so ago but failed because, though I was running wild at the time, I had not been in trouble with the police, was not playing around with men, and was at home every night. So he could do nothing . . . For years he had been treating me brutally and he feared that mother would consult the police, or a doctor on account of his incestuous behaviour towards me. So he told the doctor at the Reception House his own faults projecting them on to me and I was declared insane after being asked two questions.[14]

Was this the reason Bee had been questioning her parents so insistently about sex, despite their obvious discomfort? Was she, then a sexually immature teenager, trying to establish whether her father's constant focus was predatory and sexual as well as violent?

It is impossible to know how valid these accusations of incest are or even if Bee spoke about them with any of the examining doctors. William claimed that his daughter had a fixation on him in the letters he wrote to the Reception House when she was first committed and on later occasions, but the possibility of incest, or any kind of fixation, is not mentioned in the case notes. More than likely, any allegations by his daughter would have been assessed through prevailing views about young women's repressed sexual desires. These ideas ran in tandem with an increasing anxiety about women's growing mobility. Young, single women in the 1920s, with their increased educational and employment opportunities, began to challenge ideas about female sexuality, both in their dress and their movement into domains traditionally occupied by men. In response, popular tabloids such as *Truth* ran a series of articles on the spate of 'allegations of incest, rape and indecent assault' on defenceless men because of the 'worthless flappers' deviant, precocious proclivities'. The flapper—mobile, visible and sexual—was 'in need of rigorous control'.[15] In the eyes of social and moral reformers, genuine cases of incest were more likely to occur in overcrowded, working-class families.[16] Even then, although specific legislation had been introduced to criminalise incest in the late nineteenth century, many cases never made it to court and of those who were convicted, perpetrators often received lenient sentences.[17] Bee would also have been aware the impact such accusations would have had on her siblings and their ability to 'make suitable marriages', if her father was prosecuted,[18] along with the fact that she was dependent on him financially.

Whether it was physical or sexual, for Bee her father's behaviour was obsessive and abusive. She wrote about it in the opening pages of her first unpublished manuscript, 'Prelude to Freedom', and made oblique references in later published interviews, though she never spoke about it publicly until the months before her death: 'I didn't know then what I know now ... the truth about my father ... that he was incestuous, had a strong fixation on me. He accused me of his own fault, he said I had fixation on him.'[19]

———

After spending three days at the Reception House, on 5 December Bee was moved to Gladesville Mental Hospital. Throughout her three-and-a-half years of confinement in various mental hospitals across the state, Bee kept detailed diary notes that she later rewrote with the aim of publication. The manuscripts, titled variously 'Prelude to Freedom' and 'Advance Australia Fair', are a rich, compelling and at times poignant account of life inside four different psychiatric facilities: Gladesville, Callan Park, Kenmore and Parramatta mental hospitals. Bee was moved between these institutions as the hospital authorities sought to either 'cure' or 'punish' her, depending on her behaviour. For most of the period, she was a keen chronicler of daily life in some of the worst refractory wards, where she was often placed and, in the beginning, saw herself as an observer rather than a patient. In the opening pages of her manuscript, she describes the scene from the window of her ward at Gladesville Hospital:

> The windows of the dormitory overlook the courtyard of Ward 5. I stand on the back of a bed and gaze at the magnificent jacaranda tree which fills the centre garden. Mauve flowers, green leaves and a grey sky, what an idea for an outfit. Shall ask Aunt Ellie to buy me some grey linen for a frock, some green silk for underclothes and a piece of mauve linen for a belt . . . Anyway, though I am surrounded by faeces, what do I care? I have come from home where such things have not even been imagined and the new experience is not going to do me any harm.[20]

Bee suffered from a skin disease for most of her life. This might be why she wanted linen and silk. Clothing, and her refusal to conform to acceptable feminine dress codes, was to be an ongoing source of conflict during her confinement and was often cited as an example of her erratic behaviour. Despite her father's belief that the way she dressed was evidence of her insanity, she placed enormous significance on what she wore and understood the political and social messages certain wardrobe choices carried. It was an art form she would come to perfect in the following decades. Her aunt did send the jacaranda-inspired material to the hospital, and its theft, shortly after it arrived, caused Bee extreme distress. The theft of patients' property by staff was a constant problem that Bee bitterly resented. Regardless, her own clothing was confiscated, and she wore the same smocks as the other patients.

On her arrival at Gladesville, after three 'inert days' at the Reception House, Bee had been put to bed for a week, possibly for observation, an act she found completely irrational: 'How they expected an energetic, mentally alert girl to react to such idiotic treatment I do not know.'[21] Whatever the rationale was, she refused to comply and kept getting out of bed and demanding her clothing. This produced a response that Bee would find extremely useful over the next three years. Refusal to comply with instructions led to being sent to areas where patients were more volatile—the refractory wards. Bee thought that she was being sent there by the nurses in the hope that some of the more violent patients might attack her. In fact, it was Bee who often provoked the fights as a way of breaking the monotony of daily routines:

> I sit up in bed and keep a wary eye on Ellen while provoking her into violent action with my tongue . . . With a bound she is out of bed and stamping toward me. I dive under mine. Ellen throws it on its side but before she can do any damage to me I have caught her by the ankles and with a heave from me and a squeal from her, the floor gets a terrific bump from her buttocks. I grab her hair as she sits sprawling on the floor and that's the end. After extracting solemn promises from her I let her go. She weeps back to bed and I feel greatly eased.[22]

Physical strength was important for Bee throughout her life and she often weaponised it. At the time of her committal, she was in peak physical condition and regularly engaged in fights with both patients and nurses as a way of establishing her status as 'cock of the ward'. Sometimes it would take five nurses to subdue her. Despite her pride in her own physical strength, Bee soon noticed that the way the other female patients used their bodies was different from anything she had ever seen before, and she became fascinated by their ability to disrupt the hospital's routines and sense of female decorum:

> Much to the nurses' discomforture [sic] I do not object in the least to sleeping in the noisy end of 3. I enjoy the

movement, the colour, the uproariousness, if the day has been monotonous the night never is. Lil is very amusing. She sings obscene songs. Upon occasions she like Miss W., divests herself of her clothing and discloses a fat undulating body, as likely as not showing signs that a menses is in progress, which she parades round the dormitory while she yells her songs at the top of her voice. One that I enjoy hugely commences 'on the twenty-fourth of May, I laid her in the hay . . .' and continues erotically.[23]

During the early twentieth century women were more likely than men to be admitted into psychiatric care by the request of their spouses or family. And once admitted, their diagnoses were also more likely to have been assigned a biological basis.[24] Although the psychiatric approach was still largely somatic, men's committals were often traced to temporary economic crises or alcohol-induced delusions, which resulted in shorter committal periods (particularly after the development of Reception Houses). In the early twentieth century women, too, were seen as susceptible to external influences, particularly to the 'shocks of modernity', but primarily because of their essentially emotional dispositions, which made them vulnerable to the 'excessive energies of the modern world'. Women were believed to have a more limited physical capacity than men and more 'unstable' nervous systems.[25] Although attention had moved to the brain, psychiatric theory also sustained a link between menstruation and insanity, and claimed that women's innately nervous disposition became manifest at three crucial stages: menstruation, childbirth and menopause.[26] Psychiatrists and other medical staff were encouraged to research 'the effect of female organs, such as the ovaries, on the aetiology of female illness'.[27]

Bee and her fellow travellers in the asylums certainly fell out of the confines of acceptable female behaviour, which she described in her manuscript with meticulous and dispassionate detail. The vivid picture she paints creates a kaleidoscope of chaos, disorder and frailty, constantly breaking through the precarious layer of order imposed by the hospital's routine. In Bee's Rabelaisian portrait, women grew beards and removed their clothes at will, enthusiastically exposing menstrual blood, 'gleefully' rolling in their own excreta, and urinating freely, often for revenge against the staff,[28] all of which Bee described with a combination of scientific interest and celebration. One woman was able to squeeze milk from her breasts at least seven years after childbirth much to Bee's delighted amazement, while another claimed to have 'ninety million bums'. Mrs P, on the other hand, insisted she had divested herself of all internal organs:

> A moaning whine of 'no heart, no liver, no kidneys, no ovaries, no bowels' several times repeated . . . It is Mrs P who thinks she is dead, [and] adds 'no breadbasket'. She has to be spoon fed by several exasperated nurses who were immediately informed by her . . . that it was no use feeding her because she had no stomach. 'Where does the food go to?' asks a perspiring attendant. 'Into me bloomers!'[29]

The women often used obscene language as a form of provocation. In the Victorian era medical theory viewed this as evidence of 'women's innately immoral behaviour'.[30] Dr A.T. Edwards, who was a superintendent at Callan Park during the 1920s, had a different explanation:

> The language in the female wards was as filthy as the bodies and the beds. Probably owing to the fact that at that time women in the community led such repressed lives, in all hospitals the language in the female wards became atrocious with the removal of social restrictions, whilst in the male wards there was probably less foul language than in the general population, certainly much less than amongst the bullockies and the medical students. In the female wards

at Callan Park the female patients obviously savoured their obscene epithets with luscious enjoyment.[31]

Bee savoured them as well. Admitting that the obscenity had shocked her when she first arrived, she quickly became interested 'in the Fine Art of Swearing' and was delighted by her family's appalled reactions when she repeated choice phrases she had learned.[32] The obscenity often reflected broader social and moral judgements about women. Patients referred to each other or themselves as whores, whores' bastards, bitches or by contrast 'poor virgins' (the latter description, Bee noted, was 'gloriously' incorrect for most of the women but the 'distressing truth' about herself). At times these accusations were joyfully hurled as provocation but sometimes they played out with quiet poignancy:

> We both have affection for f. [sic] especially since her apology to the quasi-bundy clock at which the nurses must register their rounds. She, like many of the patients, thinks that it's a telephone and one night Mrs L and I awoke to find F standing stark-naked in front of it saying 'I'm sorry my mother's a bloody whore.'[33]

In both her manuscripts and public speech, Bee often identified 'moral courage' as the sublime virtue, inherent in both herself and her father, yet William had been the principal actor in her committal, and she would feel the full force of his power in the coming months. It was this act—seen by her as a duplicitous betrayal—that dominated their complicated and contradictory relationship for the rest of their lives.

4

Constraint

'Repression is the cause of insanity.'

Bee Miles, 'Advance Australia Fair', p. 28

In the early decades of the twentieth century, particularly after the First World War, women had begun to enter the workforce in greater numbers—though their choice of profession remained limited. At the same time, legislation ensured that females received proportionally less wages than males.[1] Women could vote and the New South Wales *Women's Legal Status Act* (1918) gave them limited access to public office, but they could not be jurors; female magistrates were restricted to the Bench of the Children's Court.[2] As we have seen, these small gains in increased mobility and financial independence created anxiety around the potential for greater sexual freedom as well. While there was growing discussion around women's sexuality and women's right to sexual pleasure, this was largely in relation to married, not single, women. Psychiatrists had begun to use the terms 'sexual repression' and 'sexual excitement' in their diagnoses of hysteria, but medical discourse still argued that these symptoms could be cured through 'marriage and motherhood'.[3]

Bee believed that repression caused insanity. Early in her committal, she had told her doctors that she felt sexually frustrated because

42

of her 'confinement', but their responses made her understand that discussing sexual desire with her doctors would place her in the category of morally as well as mentally 'inefficient'. Her understanding was correct. There was a strong correlation between masturbation and madness.[4] Dr Edwards, writing of the same period, noted that young, single, female psychiatric patients who displayed an interest in or knowledge about sexuality were seen as mentally unstable.[5] Perhaps sensing this, Bee decided to limit her discussions about sex to just one other patient, Mrs L, with whom she had developed a kind of friendship (though, on at least one occasion, Mrs L had tried to stab her with a pair of scissors):

> I fancy my love of fighting is due to repressed sex desires. Though I am over twenty-one I am still a virgin, yet I heartily subscribe to Parolle's philosophy on virginity.[6] Sometimes I wonder whether or not it is a rational philosophy. I cannot discuss the matter with the doctors for they cannot speak of sex without shame and that makes me feel ill; now with the nurses for the same reason. So far I have only struck one patient whom I can talk of such things with. Mrs L. is my confidante, she says that my desires are perfectly natural, and sometimes, when I behave like Lil and look at the shadow of my naked body on the dormitory wall at night and decide that the outline is very pretty, Mrs L. smiles and agrees.[7]

William was sure that his daughter had not 'fallen', due to 'a lack of sexual development and her insanity generally'. In other words, Bee's behaviour was perceived to be sexually repellent.[8] At the same time her grandmother Ellen was 'always giving her money and presents in the belief that the girl might sell herself to get what she wanted' otherwise. This was not an uncommon fear amongst some sections of the middle class in response to a new generation of mobile young female consumers.[9]

William did think that his daughter had 'homosexual tendencies'; these are also mentioned in the case notes, because of Bee's habit of kissing the nurses.[10] She freely admitted that she kissed both staff and patients but insisted that this was out of spontaneous affection. Still, she was aware that her behaviour could be perceived as having sexual overtones and therefore 'deviant':

> Several of the women appear to have been gleefully rolling on their bowel excreta so a nurse has to give them a shower. But she, like the rest of her kind fears to be called homosexual or worse dares she touch a patients [sic] genitals even with a cloth; so she sends a hail across the court to me intimating that she needs my help, I don't care that people automatically think the irrational thing and am not a prude. The temperature of the water tested, off comes the patient's nightie, off comes my nightie, and in a moment, the dirt rolls into the drain.[11]

Given the gradual development of Bee's own homophobia in later years, this early indifference is interesting. But the reluctance of the nurses to have intimate physical contact with the female patients' bodies had a more pragmatic basis. As employees in a state-controlled psychiatric institution, nurses would have been aware of the genuine risks attached to being labelled lesbian—a relatively new term in the 1920s. Lesbianism was formally classified as a mental illness and women who were assertive, who avoided sexual relations with their husbands and generally refused to fit into prescribed notions of femininity were vulnerable to the consequences of psychiatric diagnosis for lesbianism or inversion. This could result in being involuntarily subjected to a range of treatments including clitoridectomy, aversion therapy or hormone therapy.[12] Bee wrote frankly about her fascination with the physical anatomy of the female patients and 'their brown wrinkled bodies', which she volunteered to bathe, stripping herself and scrubbing down a patient 'as though she were a horse', or escorting patients to the toilet and sitting on them in order to force an emission.[13] One entry in the case notes describes Bee getting a 'patient to go down on her hands and knees and would sit on her back as though riding a pony'.[14]

Bee's public flirtations with the male doctors and brief physical encounters with a young carpenter, whom, she said, 'kissed beautifully', were also recorded in her journal with much pride. What is omitted is her seduction by a nurse, which she later claimed was a natural outcome 'when women are thrown back upon each other for any erotic stimulation'.[15] While her homoerotic behaviour did not appear to have serious ramifications during her time in New South Wales mental hospitals, it did cause potential problems in Melbourne when she was briefly confined at Royal Park Receiving House several years later.[16]

What the case notes do describe, with increasing exasperation, is Bee's complete lack of inhibition regarding her own body and sense of female decorum. Some of these complaints are relatively minor, regarding her having bare legs or wearing slippers instead of shoes. Others describe her habit of appearing with 'the scantiest of clothing', sometimes in a towel, but more often naked—particularly in the dining room. This echoes the frustration her father had expressed in his letters to the hospital regarding her refusal to wear anything but the slightest of clothing and the way it had caused major disturbances in the family home. Whether Bee's insistence on removing her clothing was due to her skin irritations or a lack of inhibition because of encephalitis lethargica is unclear. It could have been a combination of both. But it also served to usurp the order of the hospital and her insistence on parading naked during mealtimes was probably deliberate. Psychiatric hospitals placed a special focus on the dining room as a place for rehabilitation— a way for patients to be reintroduced to civilised behaviour.[17] It was also, Bee frequently noted, intensely tedious:

Everything goes smoothly until E. who is suicidal to the nth degree, throws herself backward over the form she's sitting on and cuts her scalp. I gaze awfully . . . though the excitement is welcomed. Nurses dash about, one runs for the doctor, two hold her to prevent her banging her head against the floor. She is quiet after her head has been stitched but they are taking no chances so she is tied to a form with a strong strap passed around her body.[18]

Using the female body to usurp order was a lesson Bee would never forget and she would employ it throughout her long career in public disruption. But for now, within the confines of the asylum, she would learn that the body—her source of rebellion—would also be a focus of punishment:

There is continual talk of disciplining the patients. It is not only my belief but the belief of every man and woman who understands himself that repression is the cause of insanity. Yet disciplining continues ad nauseam and ad absurdum. As a matter of fact the doctors, being only mental doctors have a sense of inferiority and exercise what power they have to the utmost. They treat us like criminal lunatics.[19]

This inherent link between criminality and insanity in judicial and medical systems, so astutely grasped by Bee in her journal, was deeply ingrained in modern liberal democracies. If individual freedom was an intrinsic citizenship right, then its removal became the ultimate punishment. Problem populations like the insane or the criminal were managed by 'a dovetailing of medical and penal' powers.[20] In the context of colonial and then post-Federation Australia, criminality and insanity had a long and tangled history. Initially, there was no separation between those deemed insane and the broader prisoner population, but the gradual influence of the British moral therapy model and sustained campaigns by the medical profession saw the introduction of Reception Houses attached to courthouses through the 1868 *Lunacy Reception Act*. At the same time, successive *Lunacy Acts* broadened grounds of arrest to include 'vagrant' and 'not under proper care'.[21]

But it was the New South Wales *Police Offences Act* (1902) that really increased police powers over the suspected insane by removing the requirement for proof of intent. This meant that the police, along with magistrates, had been awarded the power to make and enforce moral judgements on individual behaviour, particularly if that behaviour played out in public space.[22] These increased powers, for example, were used relentlessly in the continued arrests and confinements of William Chidley. With his Grecian tunic, vegetarian diet and published theories on what he believed were less aggressive forms of penetrative sex, Chidley was frequently arrested and institutionalised despite public protest. Dr Chisholm Ross, the psychiatrist who had examined Bee, was often instrumental in committing Chidley, who eventually died in Callan Park ten years before Bee was transferred there in February 1926.[23]

When the family learned that Bee was to be transferred, William wrote to the superintendent. He wanted to know what kind of treatment was being provided for his daughter and if they had given her a diagnosis, as he said none had been mentioned. The superintendent at Gladesville wrote back to inform him that 'apart from enforced restraint', Bee had not received any medical treatment and that he doubted whether 'any treatment would have been of much benefit'.[24] The family were not in favour of moving Bee from Gladesville, but the hospital made it clear that the decision had been made.

Although she disliked Callan Park more than Gladesville, particularly because female patients were not allowed to smoke, Bee did encounter a doctor there with whom she developed a positive relationship. The unnamed female doctor would bring Bee to her room and encourage her to talk about herself, a subject Bee acknowledged she found very interesting. Normally cynical about medical intervention, she thought the doctor so 'decent' that she began to confide in her, though the nature of the conversations is not recorded in the case notes. Instead, Bee's own journal noted: 'After a year's observation of insanity I have come to the conclusion that I am not mad and am beginning to long very heartily for my liberty.'

During her stay at Callan Park, Bee continued to record her experiences in her journal, where images of penal servitude and corporeal punishment begin to dominate her writing:

> I feel the loss of my liberty but am happy-natured enough to bear my imprisonment with reasonable equanimity . . . I am very resilient though brutal squashings by nurses, with or without provocation, are frequent. One nurse who had boasted high and low that she could break me . . . had me put into muffs. But I have small hands and was loose very soon . . . Some days ago I was concerned with a minor row in the laundry. I was dragged back to the ward by four nurses, who with Charge's help tried to lock me in a cell. Believing them to be unjust I resisted their efforts for about ten minutes at the end of which time Charge, dripping with perspiration, strangled me unconscious three times with her fingers, an agonizing method; a stocking is not so painful; indeed is rather pleasant . . . She hit me with her keys and turned to the other nurses saying 'come away from her girls, she's rotten with the pox.'[25]

The mental hospital system often imposed a regime of microscopic control over the most basic human activities. This became particularly difficult for Bee when she was transferred in May 1926 to Kenmore Hospital at Goulburn. Despite the onset of winter, her doctors at Callan Park believed that the change to a rural environment might improve her condition:

Two days after I arrived at this country hospital, I asked one of the doctors whether or not I might be allowed to use my tooth-brush, nail brush and other toilet articles. Why I should have to ask for them is beyond me. However the doctor said 'yes' and added 'now I hope you'll show yourself worthy of these privileges'. In every Mental Hospital we patients are treated as criminals and rights were called privileges. On entering all our possessions were taken from us.[26]

Erving Goffman, in his seminal work on total institutions (most notably the penal institution, the prisoner-of-war camp and the mental asylum), describes the way in which incarceration violates the sense of self that individuals have constructed in the everyday world. Building an alternative world around the patient, stripping them and then introducing rights or 'privileges' are 'perhaps the most important feature of inmate culture'. They create, Goffman argues, absolute dependence on an external authority. Asking permission to read or move is a process of powerlessness.[27]

Kenmore was cold. With her reputation preceding her, Bee was placed in the refractory ward upon her arrival in case she tried to escape. At night her cell was freezing and water trickled down the walls. Dr Gordon Moffitt, the superintendent, had very fixed ideas about patient treatment. His belief that animal protein was a cause of human aggression meant that patients in the refractory wards were subject to a strict vegetarian diet. Bee described the way the smell of roast meat would waft in from the neighbouring ward, causing the patients to moan with hunger. Ironically, she noted that the 'most violent patient I have met is in this vegetarian ward'. Moffitt scrutinised every aspect of patients' lives, including Bee's, censoring the books her grandmother sent to ensure they were suitable. Although Moffitt appeared to run a tightly controlled system, testimony by former patients at the 1923 Lunacy Commission revealed a harsh and chaotic environment, with drunken doctors, and frequent brutality by the staff. The food was appalling: 'It was a common occurrence to find livestock in the meat'. Bee might have been more fortunate than she knew to be in the vegetarian ward.[28]

Bee recorded the physical punishments meted out by the nurses for seemingly minor infringements in graphic detail, the telltale bruises being explained away as fights with other patients. The most frequent punishment was enforced inertia. It was a regular routine in Callan Park, where Bee returned in September 1926, for patients to have their meal tickets marked as violent, which meant they were subject to extreme levels of inactivity in the refractory wards for extended periods of time. Patients could be restrained by being strapped to seats (the straps concealed from view) or by being placed in straitjackets:

> In the hospitals I have been in most of the patients are forced to sit down all day long. It is easier for the nurses to keep an eye on them . . . One woman has been tied to a seat for at least three months and her buttocks are covered in boils. Another woman has been in a straight jacket [sic] every daytime for three years . . . A woman was confined in a straight jacket [sic] night and day for at least seven weeks. Those boiling days of summer must have nearly killed her . . . in the morning her body was in a state beyond description.[29]

Dr Edwards' recollections of Callan Park in the 1920s are strikingly similar to Bee's descriptions, though rather more poetic:

> The two female refractory wards . . . formed a reeking, malodorous oven in the summer and in the winter were like Dante's Hell of Ice. If the weather was wet or extremely cold, the patients spent the whole day, sometimes for weeks on end in complete idleness . . . The amount of sedatives and hypnotics needed to enforce twenty-four hours of . . . inactivity and sleep was tremendous . . . Some eighty to a

hundred patients a week spent many hours in seclusion in
locked single rooms or in restraint, mainly in a camisole,
a tough harsh canvas jacket … Many unfortunates spent
weeks on end in either seclusion or restraint.[30]

If we consider the architecture of the asylums where Bee was a
patient, with their grand Victorian structures, ample lands and
fruit and vegetable gardens, such as Gladesville and Callan Park in
Sydney, we can see the physical embodiment of the ideas of moral
therapy that were a feature of the nineteenth-century approach to
treating the insane. Developed by Quakers like Samuel Tuke and
other leading reformers, the principles of moral therapy involved
offering a refuge to patients from the pressures of an increasingly
industrialised world. Patients could be restored to good mental
health through daily routines of physical work, exercise and religious instruction. Even the boundaries that separated the patient
from the outside world were hidden by a ha-ha wall, a deep trench
in the ground that surrounded the asylum and was concealed within
the landscape.[31]

By the 1920s things had changed. The asylums were overcrowded
and understaffed.[32] Psychiatric practice, already a low-prestige spe-
cialty, had become dominated by the notion of heredity causes for
insanity, which led to the categorisation of curable and incurable. It
would appear that Bee had been placed in the incurable category, as
she was moved from hospital to hospital, her enforced inertia and
regime of restraint increasingly severe. In his memoirs Dr Edwards
noted the unwillingness of senior medical surgeons to perform
remedial procedures on psychiatric patients and the refusal of many
to use anaesthetics in the belief that insane patients did not feel
pain. The common response was: 'Why waste the time. He is only
a lunatic.'[33] Bee's own experiences confirm this indifference. After
being transferred from Gladesville to Callan Park, she fell seriously
ill. Her condition was met initially with apathy and then violence:

To-day I have been here three months and feel very ill . . .
lie on the court in the sun in a state of stenosis. I have a
prolapsed rectum, but something else is wrong too. I am
to be removed to Ward 2 because Charge here loathes me
and has told Super wild and lying tales to rid herself of me.
She is all sorts of a cow and the change is welcome. K— is
Charge of 2, and is a motherly looking woman . . . Motherly-
looking is all K— is. Actually she is almost as brutal as my
Charge in the first hospital. The prolapse makes it very
uncomfortable for me to use the lavatory so I asked for a
rubber receptacle in my cell. Charge wasn't having any and
punched me in the stomach to make me sit on the lavatory
seat . . . I am still ill and have no strength other than to crawl
on to the court and lie in a bed there all day. Doctor looks in
at me and orders me to sick bay.[34]

Bee later claimed that had it not been for the intervention of her
aunt in sending in the family physician, she might have died. She
spent six weeks recovering in hospital from a combination of a
prolapsed rectum and nephritis. (In fact she would suffer from
a prolapsed rectum for the rest of her life and, when she died in
1973, carcinoma of the rectum was listed as a cause of death.)[35]
Back at Callan Park, after enduring a difficult winter at Kenmore,
Bee was facing an uncertain future. There was no diagnosis and
certainly no plans for her release. The only constant was the endless
routine of inertia, boredom, violence and punishment. But when
the longed-for circuit-breaker finally came, it was through tragic
circumstances.

5

Flight

'The medicos agree I'm unaltered—why they don't say "unalterable" and call it a day is beyond me.'

Bee Miles, 'Advance Australia Fair', p. 31

In 1925, during the second year of Bee's committal, her mother fell ill. William had taken the family on a European tour and Maria became seriously unwell in Italy. Bee's initial committal notes mention that her mother was already suffering from kidney disease. William may have taken her away in the hope that travel might restore her health, or perhaps it was a desire to escape the domestic dramas that had dominated their lives for the past decade. Bee received a postcard from Italy stating that her mother was unwell and the family was returning home. Within a month of their arrival, on Armistice Day, 11 November 1925, Maria was dead. William had refused to allow his daughter to return home to see her mother in her final days.[1]

Up to this time Bee been allowed out of the hospital grounds on occasional day passes, usually in the company of girlfriends. During one of these occasions, when she went out with a friend, Bee had gone to her grandmother's house in Strathfield. Her father called the hospital, which sent an escort to bring her back. She apparently came willingly and returned without incident, which was recorded in her case notes.

But there is another incident, which was later described in a sensational article in *Smith's Weekly*. Sometime during October 1925, Bee had met up with a subeditor from a literary magazine on one of her day passes. (It is not clear how long she had known him, but the notes from her initial committal at the Reception House mention that she had met someone she liked.) Soon after her trip to the city, the subeditor arranged to escort her on another day pass from Callan Park. He took her to a Registry Office in the city to organise a marriage—perhaps as a way of securing her permanent release. Somehow the family were alerted and 'at the critical moment' one of her brothers—probably John—burst in citing 'just cause and impediment' as a reason to interrupt the service. The couple was escorted to the family solicitor's office, where William was waiting. Bee was returned to Callan Park. Nothing was recorded in her patient notes, and she never mentioned it in her writing.[2]

Back in hospital, Bee immediately began planning another escape. She tried convincing her subeditor to take part in a new plan by impersonating her brother, but he was reluctant, having been threatened with imprisonment after their failed marriage bid. Whether she found help elsewhere is unclear, but in January 1926 she escaped again, this time for longer. She managed to get to Queensland, where some of her mother's family still lived. Her father placed daily advertisements in the *Daily Telegraph*, discreetly adding she was 'missing from home' and had last been seen, dressed in black, in Pitt Street.[3] He also placed notices in the *Police Gazette*, listing her as a 'missing friend'.[4] Although Bee was absent for three weeks, Callan Park did not seem overly anxious to locate her. In the end she was betrayed by someone who alerted the Queensland police. Little is known about how she survived during this period, but somehow she managed to obtain three independent diagnoses from psychiatrists who declared her 'peculiar' but not insane. She was brought back to Sydney at the instigation not of the hospital but of her father.

Although she was now in possession of three independent psychiatric assessments, Bee was again returned to Callan Park, where despite the seemingly nonchalant attitude towards her escape, her confinement and treatment became more severe. Subject to ten days of 'solitary' confinement, the case notes refer to her as 'a regular source of trouble, restless, exuberant, impulsive, imperious, violently resists . . . has had a day in seclusion'.[5] The result of this rebellion was an endless series of transfers between institutions and refractory wards with increasing inertia through medication and physical restraint, where she was faced with growing animosity from the staff:

> Here I am back again. Charges have been shifted and . . .
> that dirty vain woman, who revelled in her lousy ward when
> I first came in, bosses over me once more. Her dislike of me
> is even more marked and she badgers me incessantly and
> tells such appalling lies of me that I spend most of my days
> in a cell while she purloins my treasures. The strain of living
> under unpleasant conditions is beginning to tell on me. One
> day I am transferred to Ward 4 and for a week am kept under
> confinement, saturated with powders and cerebral sedatives.
> I am going to be sent to another hospital and this is Super's
> method of preparing the body for execution.[6]

The nurses' resentment towards their patient might have been due to an incident earlier when Bee first came to Callan Park. Bed bugs were legion and attacked the patients' flesh, particularly at night. Bee had complained to the matron, who ignored her until she reported it directly to the doctor. Though the bugs were treated and temporarily exterminated, they quickly returned, and Bee was punished for raising the complaint.[7]

Shortly after her transfer to Ward 4, Bee was moved to Parramatta Mental Hospital, which she claimed was the worst hospital she had experienced in her three years of 'imprisonment'. She thought that the superintendent suffered from 'extreme sexual repression'. What he thought of his new patient is unrecorded, but he put Bee under close observation for a week. She found the inertia impossible and began to pace the ward. In response she was refused any reading material, placed in a straitjacket and put in a cell. As soon as she was released, she orchestrated her move to the worst refractory ward, where once more, the theatre of chaos was a welcome relief from the boredom. There she was treated a little more humanely by the charge nurse who allowed her to have some of her books, only to be told by the superintendent that her choice of literature was too 'heavy' for her. She also recorded one of the worst incidents of brutality she had ever witnessed by a nurse against a patient. The patient had been given a large dose of castor oil and in retaliation had thrown a bucket of water over the nurse. Outraged, the nurse dragged the patient to the floor by her hair and assaulted her. When the super-intendent questioned the patient's bruising, the nurse said she'd been attacked by another patient. No further action was taken.[8]

Bee had been at Parramatta for two months when, one night in February 1927, she put into action another escape plan. She had at some point discovered that she was able to fit through an open space between the top of the door and the ceiling. Now she crept down the passage, avoiding patients who might raise the alarm if they spied her. She made it into the courtyard after borrowing some street clothes from another patient and narrowly avoided being spotted by a nurse, who suddenly emerged from a doorway. Dragging a garden bench to the boundary, she jumped one fence, then another and finally a third, and then she was out.

This time Bee headed for Melbourne where she was joined by her erstwhile subeditor. They took refuge in a boarding house but it wasn't long before her lack of decorum—which included smoking, loud arguments with her companion and shoeless visits to the bathroom—caused her to be reported to the police.[9] She was arrested and taken to Royal Park Receiving House. Police in

Sydney had already been alerted to her escape and arrest warrants had been issued.[10] She was returned to Parramatta Mental Hospital, but not before her appearance in the Melbourne Magistrates' Court had caught the attention of *Smith's Weekly*, and it was to their offices that she returned several weeks later after escaping for a third and final time with help from the paper's staff, who relished the fact that they had 'sprung her from the rat house'.[11]

If *The Bulletin* was the 'bushman's friend' then *Smith's* was the digger's. Established by James Joyton Smith, the venerable Claude McKay and Robert Clyde Packer (grandfather of Kerry), it attracted many fine writers and black-and-white illustrators over its long life, including Ken Slessor, Elizabeth Riddell, Lenny Lower, George Finey, Stan Cross and Rosaleen Norton (later known as the Witch of the Cross). Although it specialised in sensational headlines and scandals, it also had a strong penchant for a crusade—particularly on behalf of those the paper believed to be vulnerable. People locked away in mental asylums against their will through the machinations of family members was a favourite hobby horse of more salacious publications like *Truth* and tapped into a common public anxiety about the increasing power of the medical profession—with the memory of Chidley still very much in the public's mind. *Smith's* had higher journalistic standards than *Truth*, but the editors could recognise a sensational story when they saw one.[12]

Bee was taken across the border to Queensland under the watchful eye of *Smith's* private detective and occasional journalist John O'Donnell, with a female staff member acting as chaperone.[13] Then on 19 March 1927 the paper issued a front-page story with a screaming headline: 'Madhouse Mystery of Beautiful Sydney Girl'. The article described Bee as a 'beautiful vivacious Sydney girl of education and refinement' condemned to a lifetime 'in a madhouse' by a 'routine police court verdict'. But more damaging for William was the veiled hint of something darker: 'And behind the obvious tragedy a strange background of battle between opposing wills, the true history of which may never be told.'[14]

William, who had been more than reckless in his role as a political agitator in the past, was not prepared to have his domestic life
paraded in public. He issued a writ for libel against the paper for
£10,000, which received even more publicity as it was widely reported
on by *Smith's* rival newspapers. This was a substantial amount—
around one million dollars in today's money. William appears to
have been willingly assisted by Dr Moffitt, the superintendent of
Kenmore, who provided statements from nurses about Bee's erratic
behaviour to William's lawyer, along with his own emphatic conclusion: 'I am of the opinion that she was insane while she was here and
required to be kept in order like a child.'[15]

This was enough for the paper to offer to settle before court and
to issue an apology in their August issue. But it was also enough
for William to concede that he would be unlikely to 'put her away
again'.[16] Instead, he gave his daughter an allowance of £3 10 shillings a week, around the same wage as a bootmaker or a hairdresser.
Much to the amusement of Slessor and the dismay of the proprietors,
Bee promptly set up camp in the corridors of *Smith's*. As Slessor later
observed, the paper couldn't evict her because the whole point of the
original article was that 'she was sane'.[17]

The question remains, had Bee not secured her own release in
such dramatic and public circumstances, would she have remained
under involuntary psychiatric care for the remainder of her life?
Letters from her father and brother to the hospital superintendents
at Gladesville and Kenmore don't inquire about a potential release.
In 1926 Bee's brother John wrote to Dr Moffitt at Kenmore, inti-
mating that the family was in no hurry for her to return to Sydney,
having already made up their minds about Bee's mental state: 'My
father wrote to Dr Wallace recently that he regarded Beatrice as
seriously and permanently insane. I entirely agree with that.'[18]

It is only in the correspondence from Bee's grandmother Ellen
that there is a sense of genuine concern for her welfare, her physical
health and her potential release. It is clear from the letters that there
is tension between William, John and the grandmother, particularly

over the money Ellen was sending her granddaughter. From his earliest communications with the Reception House, William asked that his mother Ellen be 'kept out of touch, personally or by letter'.[19] Corresponding with Moffitt in June on behalf of his father, John asked to be kept informed if 'if any other money has been sent to you for her and by whom it was sent'.[20] A month later Moffitt received £3 from Bee's grandmother. This was double the amount her father was sending for her expenses. Ellen asked that the payment not be disclosed 'to any other member of my family'.[21] Bee later claimed that it was only through her grandmother's intervention that her father eventually agreed to provide her with a weekly allowance after the *Smith's Weekly* case. Her only other consistent support came from her Aunt Ellie, her grandmother's cousin. Although she was aged over eighty and had to travel a considerable distance, Aunt Ellie visited Bee regularly, sent her gifts (like the material that was stolen) and would have given her money to facilitate her escape if she hadn't been so afraid of Bee's father.

Bee claimed that the hospitals never provided genuine evidence of her insanity, and this is borne out in the case notes, which do not contain a firm diagnosis. But what is clear is that, from very early in Bee's committal, doctors had come to the conclusion that treatment was pointless. The hospital's reluctance to pursue her after her escapes, and the relief they expressed when she was moved on, indicate that she was probably not viewed as dangerous, yet she was involuntarily readmitted and subjected to increasingly severe treatment on each occasion.

The length of Bee's initial confinement (three-and-a-half years) and the draconian response to her resistance through the use of social isolation and chemical and physical restraint was similar to that of other women who were confined with her.[22] Many of these women appear to have been long-term residents and Bee only mentions the release of one patient. Most of the women were not destined to return to their communities. The gradual reforms that eventually led to the *Richmond Report* in 1983, which saw the closure of the grand asylum buildings and their inevitable transformation into luxury apartments for aspiring urban dwellers—including the Darlinghurst Reception House—were unimaginable in the 1920s.

Bee's continued insistence that she had been wrongfully detained also spoke to a broader social concern regarding the increased power of doctors over the personal freedom of individuals. The expansion of asylums in the late nineteenth century fanned public anxiety about wrongful incarceration and the motivation of the psychiatric profession. Groups such as the Lunacy Reform League, later known as the Citizen's Liberty League, generated significant amounts of adverse publicity about dubious committals into psychiatric care. Two of the league's most vocal members were the Gullett sisters, who were also members of the New South Wales Shakespeare Society along with William Miles. Their successful lobbying eventually led to the 1923 Royal Commission into Lunacy Law and Administration, which was the most extensive inquiry of its kind until the 1960s.[23] It was the same anxiety that *Smith's* capitalised on in the article that did, in the end, secure Bee's freedom.

Yet despite the intensity of the league's activities, the Royal Commission largely exonerated psychiatric practice. Some of the most supportive statements regarding the quality of care came from members of the Board of Official Visitors.[24] Introduced under Section 86 of the *Lunacy Act*, the Board was a means of allaying public anxiety about patient welfare due to the potential for abuse in isolated and autonomous asylums. Along with official visitors, feminists had also lobbied to have female protectors introduced into both prisons and psychiatric institutions.[25] Bee thought they were a decorous and useless prop:

> This is the afternoon for the Board ladies to make their
> sacred and silent appearance. They tiptoe . . . through the
> refractory wards with fear on their faces. Sister and a couple
> of nurses form their bodyguard. I have not yet found the

actual use for these women but wish Mrs L. would go for one of them. They're so respectable that a good scragging [sic] might make them a bit more human. I think they are here to see that no person is wrongfully incarcerated but . . . they are in the hands of Super who just falls short of telling them what they must think.[26]

In the late nineteenth and early twentieth centuries wrongful incarceration had been a middle-class concern. By the 1920s the medical profession had gained greater control in the discourse of efficiency and scientific management of the 'unfit' and groups like the league—characterised as largely female and eccentric—were even more marginalised.[27] Although Bee's manuscript was written in this climate, it is difficult to imagine her joining a movement, particularly a marginalised one comprised of feminists, socialists and theosophists, who were motivated by reform.

Instead, Bee's experiences as a psychiatric patient were influential in the formation of her fundamental belief that the individual was engaged in a constant battle against an irrational social order: the 'arbitrary assumptions or authority' that rationalists rejected. It became the marker against which she set her lifelong pursuit of individual freedom. The intrinsic rights of citizenship (and the framework of liberal progressivism)—self-determination, autonomy and freedom: rights that had been removed when she was institutionalised—became the metaphorical and actual cornerstones of her future transgressions. 'When constituted authority comes into conflict with an unauthorised person', she observed, 'believe the unauthorised person.'[28]

Bee's record of her three-year committal—'Prelude to Freedom'—is a portrait of oppression and power, focused on the treatment of female psychiatric patients. Within its pages Bee casts herself as an observer, though she clearly feels a sense of solidarity with these women and celebrates their minor acts of rebellion and their anarchy. Over the next decade, however, she would shift and move increasingly towards a type of nationalism that embraced many of the ideas she had originally rejected. She would come to see women, through a perceived lack of agency, as 'weak creatures' and the reforming nature of feminism as futile. During the nineteen thirties, in a period where ideological groups merged and overlapped, adapting and exploiting each other's rhetoric to consolidate their own dominance, Bee, like her father, began to move across the dividing lines. And her struggle against state-mandated control, through the judicial system, the police, and the medical profession, would escalate.

But for the moment she was 'young and free'. She found a room in Darlinghurst and a community that seemed to accept her. And for the following decade, in cities and towns across the country, she became spectacular.

6

Adventures in Bohemia

'Bea Miles, then like Lil Abner's girl, shapely and brown in shorts far ahead of their time . . .'

Kenneth Slessor, 'My Kings Cross', *Bread and Wine: Selected Prose*

Bee once described her life from the age of 25 as the beginning of her 'sylvan existence'. The campaign by *Smith's Weekly* to secure her freedom had been a success and would be proudly recalled over the years by many of the newspaper's former staff. These accounts omit the public apology *Smith's* was forced to issue to her father in its August edition and the out-of-court settlement they had reached. This was not such a major event for its publishers, who claimed to have spent £50,000 in defence costs in the paper's first five years of publication.[1] It would have been far more galling for them to admit that less than a month after her sensational rescue, their 'madhouse beauty' was once again a patient in a psychiatric institution and that she was there as a voluntary patient. On 12 April 1927 Bee entered Bayview House at Tempe.[2] Bayview was a private psychiatric hospital overlooking the Cooks River. It was marketed to prospective patients and their families who found the public system 'repulsive to their feelings' and had the financial means to pay for their care. It is not clear why Bee had become a voluntary patient so soon after her much-celebrated escape from Parramatta, or who was paying for her care, but her decision could have had a purely pragmatic basis. Winter was approaching fast, and she couldn't continue to camp in the corridors of *Smith's* offices indefinitely. Perhaps her father's allowance had not yet been finalised. Rather than risk being arrested for vagrancy, and then almost certainly taken back to the Reception House, she could voluntarily submit to psychiatric care and then be free to leave when it suited. Her eventual exit from Bayview is not recorded, but she was still there in August when her father was enjoying the public apology issued by *Smith's*.

———

By 1928 Bee was circulating in public and revelling in her freedom. She was boarding at a private residence in Chatswood on Sydney's North Shore and visiting the beach at Manly every day. But in what was to become a regular pattern, ordinary pursuits always contained an element of risk, and were guaranteed to attract the attention of the authorities. On this occasion it was the beach inspectors and the entire municipal council. Bee's transgressions consisted of swimming out half a kilometre from the shoreline and then embarking on a swim from South Steyne to Queenscliff and back; a distance of around four-and-a-half kilometres. This was considered dangerous enough—and further, they claimed, than any man had ever swum—but it was the fact that, when other swimmers tried to emulate her, they had to be rescued that really caused consternation for the beach inspectors. On the day a reporter from *Truth* arrived on the beach to investigate the story, two swimmers had already been retrieved from the surf. The large knife that Bee carried, suspended by a belt from her waist, was also causing some anxiety. She insisted that it was for pricking 'blue bottles' and protecting her if she were attacked by a shark. The knife had been seized and was being held by Manly police, while members of Manly Council considered their options. But it seems the *Truth* reporter was far more interested in describing

Bee's appearance in cinematic detail as she emerged from the surf, his pen lingering over every part of her body:

> She stands up, and like Venus Anadyomene—in a green costume—emerges. The lithe, golden brown figure, well knit, athletic, but nonetheless womanly, makes its way up the golden beach . . . She looks no more than 20, is distinctively attractive, not in a conventional flapperish way, but in a way that holds interest . . . Fair hair, thoughtful forehead, broad face, high cheekbones, firm chin, firm mouth—but nothing mean about it—nose slightly retrousse, athletic figure, well developed. Long, pale blue eyes with a twinkle seldom far away . . . this is the girl that has all of Manly, from the mayor down, puzzled.[3]

In the article Bee spoke openly about her family background, identifying her grandmother as the famous contralto Madam Cordner-Miles, her North Shore childhood, her Irish, English and Polish heritage and her own abilities as a singer and pianist. Over time she became far more circumspect about her family when speaking to journalists, but in this early interview she was keen to establish her credentials both personally and intellectually. There was a veiled reference to her recent committals when she spoke about finally having her 'liberty' and her belief in the doctrine of 'non-interference'; her opinion on writers including George Bernard Shaw, Aldous Huxley and H.L. Mencken; and her dismissal of poetry as devoid of value when compared with truth. 'The truth is everything.'

The *Truth* reporter found it hard to conceal his astonishment at his subject's erudition: 'It is rather staggering to hear the classics quoted—word perfect—by a slip of shingled, merry, blue-eyed, shark baiting siren.' Perhaps having finally run out of adjectives, he acknowledged that: 'There is something elusive in her personality that cannot be caught on a metaphorical pin and examined.' He couldn't quite make up his mind if she was 'savage or super-cultured'.

Despite Bee claiming that she was 'heartwhole' and could go where she liked and say what she thought, the outcome of Manly Council's extraordinary meeting was to grant its lifesavers authority to ban Bee from the beach. The results were reported more prosaically in the *Women's Mirror*, though it did note that Bee was probably the only woman in Australia to have been the subject of an entire municipal council meeting. As a result of the council's decision, Bee bought a new knife and began swimming at Bondi, just a tram ride from her new home on the 'Alps' of Darlinghurst and the city, known by a select group as the 'sea coast of Bohemia'.[4]

———

In the 1920s Sydney was still a walking town with its commercial boundaries clearly defined. The ferries would spill out crowds of city workers and shoppers each morning, who would march up the slopes of streets that floated up from the harbour like tendrils. Pedestrians were kept to the left, often with a dividing line down the pavement. For newly arrived black-and-white artist George Finey, the city was laid out like a ship: 'Taking George, Pitt, Castlereagh, and Elizabeth Streets as the four masts of a sailing ship, and the other streets that cross them at right angles, Park and King amongst others as the spars of a square-rigger, with the Quay as the ship's hull, and Central Station as the masthead, you have a marine blueprint.'[5]

The shopping and commercial circuit ran from the dockside warehouses at Circular Quay to the train terminus at Railway Square. Large department stores such as Anthony Horden's, Peapes', Farmer's and Mark Foy's offered a broad selection of goods, while arcades like the Angel, the Royal, the Strand and the Victoria, running between the major streets, featured speciality shops and restaurants housed within grand Victorian facades, of which only the Strand remains. On blisteringly hot summer days, a flag would fly over the GPO at Martin Place, announcing the arrival of the southerly, which, when it came, blew welcome gusts of wind down the narrow streets. Martin Place was full of flower stalls; Sargent's pie shops dotted the landscape offering lunch for three pence. A tram ride from one end of the city to the other cost two pence.

But there was another Sydney, as there is in every city, whose geography was defined by pubs, wine shops, cheap restaurants, small struggling theatres and single rooms, where people met, wrote, painted, argued, drank and played. This was the 'sea coast of Bohemia', and it was here, for almost a decade, that Bee found solace, refuge and the kind of freedom she so desperately sought. Central Station to the west, Darlinghurst to the east and Circular Quay to the north were the borders of Bohemia with pubs and cafes spread across the city within. Its citizenry was comprised chiefly of artists, musicians and writers, who preferred the vibrancy of the city to the stultifying environment of the suburbs. There was a conscious movement away from the previous generation's nationalist iconography of the isolated bushman, as artists turned their gaze to the ever-changing, constantly moving city-scapes, and the gradual rise of the Sydney Harbour Bridge, captured so evocatively in visual works by artists like Thea Proctor and Grace Cossington Smith. Bohemia in the 1920s was represented by a Sydney-defined group of artists who celebrated the immediacy of their urban environment and lived life as an art form,[6] and this had major appeal for Bee.

Part of the bohemian vision was concerned with transplanting and revitalising European culture within a local context as a type of Australian renaissance. Classical Greek imagery was transposed onto uniquely Australian landscapes. The artist Norman Lindsay, who in turn was influenced by both Nietzsche and Plato, developed much of the guiding philosophy, embracing the notion of the artist hero. He saw the artist as the sublime individual, the embodiment of a creative force that was essentially masculine.

Bee was also influenced by Nietzsche in her later development of a hierarchy of genius, although she used intellect rather than creative talent as its defining feature. Lindsay's son Jack, classics scholar, polymath, poet and eventual Marxist, attempted to articulate bohemian artistic theory in the short-lived publication *Vision*, which he established with Kenneth Slessor and Frank Johnson and with significant support from Norman: 'If we wish to express an Australian spirit, let us make the spirit worth expressing by adding to it all the stimulus of sensuousness and lyric imagery we can, by creating beauty so that the general consciousness can be further vitalised.'[7]

Whether it was through the evocation of nymphs and satyrs frolicking on the Sydney shoreline, or through the celebration of a modern, rising, city skyline, 'Bohemian artistic vision was consciously seeking a different kind of national identity'.[8] *Vision* was launched in 1923—a fateful year for Bee. She was already mixing in literary and artistic circles before her committal and had contributed a piece of music criticism to the journal *Triad*.[9] Jack's uncle, the artist Lionel Lindsay, was well acquainted with her family and she knew his daughter Jean. One of her brothers had been Jean's first boyfriend, and both Jean and her brother Peter had visited Bee when she was in the asylums. *Smith's* had claimed that it was her early forays into bohemian life, where she 'courted the company of poets and artists', which had caused so much concern for her family and led to her committal. There was much in *Vision* that would have appealed to Bee: its aspirations to express a uniquely Australian identity fused with a radical newness, an overt sensuality, a rejection of Christianity and an impulse to shock. She had grown up in a home that embraced European philosophical and cultural traditions while actively, and often provocatively, cultivating an independent and distinctively Australian political culture. At the same time, her father's interest in botany and natural sciences had given her a love for the beauty of the local environment. Australia was not the protestant child of the British Empire but an ancient, pre-Christian landscape that was alive with sensuality and promise.

Unfortunately, *Vision*, which began with ambition and confidence, quietly folded after four issues, though its three founders went on to find success. Slessor continued to develop his poetic voice, while earning his living as a journalist and editor and was at *Smith's* during Bee's famous liberation from 'the rat house' (Parramatta Mental Hospital). Jack Lindsay eventually went to London where he became involved with Franfolico Press and was joined by another Queenslander, Percy 'Inky' Stephensen. Together they produced fine productions of Greek and Latin translations illustrated by Norman, along with the periodical *London Aphrodite*. A decade later Stephensen would embark on another national publishing project with Bee's father with very different objectives. Frank Johnson had a successful career as a publisher of Australian writing and would reappear years later in Bee's life as she continued the struggle to have her manuscripts published.

The year that Bee gained her freedom, 1927, was the height of Sydney's bohemian movement. Writer and freelance journalist Dulcie Deamer, also known as the Queen of Bohemia, called it the 'Golden Decade'. Jack Lindsay described it as 'the Roaring Twenties'. It was a parallel universe of artists, writers, poets and their supporters, working as freelancers or employed as writers, cartoonists or illustrators in one of a growing number of publications like *Smith's*. Sydney was a small and intimate city, but although everybody knew each other, not everyone frequented the same establishments, which opened and shut according to their changing fortunes. The Café La Boheme in Wilmot Street, where the poet and scholar Christopher Brennan, from an older generation of bohemians, was a frequent patron, and where his beautiful daughter Anna had famously danced on the tables, had closed but other cafes and wine shops were flourishing. The Roma in Pitt Street and Pellegrini's in the basement of 85 Elizabeth Street were establishments where Jack Lindsay often drank. Mockbell's coffee shops, where people played dominoes and chess in their lunch hours, covered the city from Circular Quay to Central. Slessor, Lindsay and Johnson met there daily while they were planning the first issue of *Vision*. In the evenings those who had money frequented the more upmarket Latin Café in the

Royal Arcade. Pubs, like the Angel, Usher's and Pfalhert's, clustered around lower George Street, catered for the journalists of *The Bulletin*, while staff from *Smith's* drank at the Assembly and the Tudor in Phillip Street. These were exclusively male drinking establishments. But for many bohemians, male and female, their universe was located in two rooms up a set of steep stairs at 219 Elizabeth Street. Pakie's Club opened on 8 June 1929 and immediately became the adopted home for aspiring and established artists and writers. It was a dry establishment—no alcohol was served—and its main fare was macaroni cheese and salads, served by the proprietor, Augusta (Pakie) Macdougall. Pakie's modernist décor was designed with the assistance of Roy De Maistre and Walter Burley Griffin. Griffin and his wife Marion were regular patrons. Pakie was close friends with the Griffins and probably introduced Marion to Bee.

The Griffins had embarked on an ambitious project to establish a residential community at Castlecrag on Sydney's lower North Shore. Houses were designed to harmonise with the local environment and were centred around communal spaces. There were no fences or boundaries to separate the buildings from the natural landscape. An amphitheatre was constructed for the many plays and performances that Marion produced. Pakie lived in one of the Griffins' houses, and members of Pakie's Club were regular weekend visitors, including Bee. She shared Marion's love of the Australian landscape, her energy and her forthrightness. Louise Lightfoot, who was the first female to graduate in architecture from the University of Melbourne, worked for the Griffins and recalled that Marion welcomed everyone 'but the only one who was perfectly free with Marion and said what she liked was the well-known eccentric character Bea Miles; and Marion appreciated her for this'.[10]

On Saturday nights members of Pakie's Club also staged theatrical and musical performances, and it was here Bee could often be found, seated at the piano, wearing a white dress draped in folds like a Corinthian column over her shoulders, playing Scarlatti. She was, in the words of one former admirer, 'beautiful'. When she wasn't playing the piano, she was at the centre of every discussion group, always—like her father—talking a little too loudly. The writer Dymphna Cusack remembered the first time she saw Bee and was 'staggered':

> She came in on a hot Saturday night, we always had a dance there; magnificent body, tall with short blonde hair and spotless white shorts and shirt and sandals . . . we didn't begin to wear shorts or slacks publicly till the end of the thirties . . . But Bee looked . . . superb . . . She struck me as being a very sensible woman in a very stupid community . . . She was far more intelligent and rational than most ordinary people you met . . . She was outspoken and utterly frank but as for any sign of mental disturbance I never saw it.[11]

George Finey was a regular at Pakie's and was also working at *Smith's* when they orchestrated Bee's final escape. He claimed that Bee had a 'cartoonist's mind', able to 'strip any subject of unwanted words and present it in a few mental brush strokes'. For Finey, she represented the 'spirt of the twenties'.[12] Pakie's clientele not only tolerated her, they actively made space for her. No one seemed to find her ideas strange, her manner 'childish' or her clothing a sign of 'madness'. She had found a world where she could finally be 'heartwhole', where she could say what she liked and people listened to her. Inside this hospitable and creative atmosphere, with Pakie as her trusted banker and friend, she could flourish. Outside its protective walls was a different story. There, the threat of arrest and re-committal was ever present and genuine.

In January 1929, six months before Pakie's had opened, Bee was arrested for 'acting in an irresponsible manner' in Darlinghurst, where she had taken a room at 58 Darlinghurst Road. According to her admission records, Bee had been riding on the bumper bars of cars and refused to see the seriousness of her behaviour:

> She is foolish and childish in her outlook. Irresponsible and
> her ideas show a lack of balance of conduct—can see no
> reason for not riding on the bumper bar of cars.[13]

The certificate was signed by Chisholm Ross, the same doctor who
had certified Bee in 1923. He resigned from the Reception House
in 1931, but at the time of Bee's 1929 admission he was still certifying patients. Unlike Bee's first admission in 1923, there was no
mention of encephalitis lethargica as a possible contributing factor
to her behaviour, although the certifying doctor stated that Bee was
well known to him. At the time of her arrest and committal Bee
was employed as a proofreader for Ross Bothers Printers in Kent
Street Sydney.[14]

Bee remained in Gladesville Psychiatric Hospital for three
months. During her stay she underwent psychological testing,
which declared her IQ 'to be 108 and her mental age to be 17 years,
4 months'. How this curiously precise age was determined is not
detailed. The case notes show that she was reasonably compliant,
though she was 'anxious for talks on philosophy or dramatic art
criticism . . . writes frequent letters—spelling occasionally wrong'.
One of these letters was to a female doctor, with whom she seemed
to have a more positive relationship:

> Dear Dr Beveridge
> Having no one to talk to here I address myself to you. This
> morning I bathed about 9 patients exclusive of myself.
> Feeling stenotic I took half a cup of that White Draught.
> Beastly stuff but it made me feel better. Mrs D is a rowdy
> brute and BA with her 'I'm not under the earth am I?' nearly
> [drove] me into a decline.[15]

After describing the routine dullness of life on the ward, Bee turned
to the subject of poetry (the value of which she had dismissed the
year before). Now she wrote in praise of the triolet—a verse form

she described as 'perfect. One sentence made up of several clauses, meaning carried into and beyond the repeated lines'. Then, in a playful, teasing manner, she questioned the lack of diagnosis for her committal: 'Am I insane? That is the question—whether 'tis nobler to be merely abnormal or, having run the gamut of the R.H. [Reception House] and Chisholm [Ross], to be widely homicidal, suicidal, paranoic, dementia precoxical . . . Perhaps I have O.P. (G.P.?) one never knows.'[16]

No one ever seemed to know. As with Bee's previous committal period at Gladesville, there was no confirmed diagnosis. Almost immediately she began a letter-writing campaign to secure her freedom, writing initially to the superintendent at Gladesville Hospital requesting release. The pianist Jascha Spivakovsky was performing a series of concerts at the Sydney Town Hall. Widely regarded as the world's greatest pianist, Spivakovsky had a hugely successful Australian concert tour in 1922, and Bee had attended his Sydney recital. In her letters she stated that she was desperate not to miss the current event and went to great lengths to explain why he was such an important musician. She wrote every week listing the dates she had missed and the ever-decreasing opportunities to hear him play. When that didn't work, she wrote about an upcoming theatrical production at the St James Theatre. The producer was Sir Benjamin Fuller, owner of the theatre and a highly successful theatrical entrepreneur. Bee claimed that he had given her permission to sit in on rehearsals as she wished to study 'stage craft with a view to becoming a dramatic critic'. She had already been writing for *The Bulletin*, *Smith's* and the *News*. She would, she guaranteed, absolutely settle down and forget her foolishness if she were allowed her freedom. Her conduct, she promised, would be 'irreproachable and of a kind befitting my years'.[17] She also wrote directly to Dr Hogg, the inspector general of mental hospitals, putting forward an argument for her release. When she had escaped from Parramatta Mental Hospital in 1927, she told him, she 'went on the loose' for two years—'not so much because I am mentally unstable, as because

I was full of the joy of being free after three years of detention'. Even though she was living in Kings Cross, 'a somewhat loose locality', she hadn't landed in any 'unpleasant situation'. Her social events were limited to evenings at the Playbox Theatre. (The Playbox, a tiny upstairs venue in Rowe Street, was run by Duncan Macdougall, Pakie's husband.) She insisted that she never entertained at home and hadn't been in trouble apart from riding bumper bars.

Bee was not the only one writing letters. William wrote to the superintendent in February to say that during her last committal Bee's repeated returns to hospital after her escapes had been at his own 'great trouble and considerable expense' and that if she escaped again, he would 'leave her to the Crown'. A few weeks later he wrote to the superintendent again, informing him that he was going to visit his daughter the following week and would like to have a meeting with the superintendent as well. He was also planning to speak with Dr Chisholm Ross. William was preparing for an extended overseas trip and would be away for six months. While in England he intended consulting 'some alienist who is knowledge-able about psychoanalysis'. It was 'most likely Beatrice had (and has) a father fixation but that fact in itself doesn't help'. He was not happy when he learned that one of the consulting doctors had concluded that Bee was not insane and began offering his own diag-noses, eventually landing on 'moral imbecility'. The superintendent disagreed and gently suggested that since William was clearly inter-ested in Freudian analysis, perhaps he should take his daughter to Europe with him to see a psychoanalyst. William was not happy with this suggestion either. He had no intention of taking his daughter anywhere. He had ceased to be surprised, he wrote, about how his daughter managed to convince people that she was not insane, adding that she had a 'kind of charm for some . . . and in some ways very clever with words. To me, however, she appears always insane . . . her hopes and expectations . . . quite imbecile'. As far as he was concerned her fate was a 'triangle of freedom, prison and mental hospital until she "goes out" with an accident'.[18]

But in March the hospital began to allow her occasional outings by herself and Bee was finally discharged as 'recovered' while on leave in June. It is unclear what 'recovered' signified, but if it meant that Bee would cease climbing onto moving cars it was grossly optimistic, despite her promises. By the late 1920s cars had become her preferred mode of transport and in Sydney, where car numbers had risen, there was a banquet of choice. In less than a decade the number of vehicles per 100 people in New South Wales had increased from two to ten.[19] When she was outside the city centre, Bee would often attempt to wave cars down for a lift, which meant the drivers who stopped chose willingly to allow her into their vehicles. Within the built-up areas of the city centre, where cars idled in traffic near pedestrians, she dispensed with any gestures towards propriety. Instead, she would climb nimbly onto the back or sideboard of a stationary or slow-moving car, occasionally resting on the spare tyre, with the driver quite often oblivious. And that was how, in the winter of 1929, she met Bernard Hesling.

Hesling, newly arrived from England, was struggling to make a living as an interior designer and set decorator. He was a stranger in Sydney and lonely for the artistic circles he had left behind in London. He first saw Bee in Macquarie Street near the Botanic Gardens and was instantly entranced by this 'faun-like' creature climbing gracefully onto the back of a Bentley, who dressed the way his friends in London did and was 'so fantastically vital, so lithe, with her boyish cropped hair, her clear-cut features . . . She wore no make-up and her face glowed with health'.[20]

After obtaining Bee's address through an acquaintance, Hesling put on his best clothes and called on Bee where she was staying at Woolloomooloo. An Indian motorbike was parked outside and Hesling soon learned that Bee was preparing to ride pillion to Brisbane with her boyfriend. After discovering that Hesling was new in Sydney and didn't know anyone, Bee took him to Pakie's, where she introduced him to the artistic community he had been seeking since he arrived. On his first night he was introduced to

Marion and Walter Burley Griffin, writers Dymphna Cusack and Kylie Tennant, and the anthropologist Professor Radcliffe Brown. (Bee had once famously told him his profession was a magnificent waste of time). Hesling also met Adela Pankhurst Walsh and her husband Tom. Adela, daughter of the suffragette Emmeline Pankhurst, would have been well known to Bee, given her close association with Bee's father during the anti-conscription campaigns a decade before. Both Adela and Tom had been leading figures in socialist campaigns and founding members of the Communist Party of Australia. Tom had been president of the Seamen's Union and led a series of national industrial action campaigns that made him an enemy of the Commonwealth Government. The latter waged its own campaign to have Walsh deported and to break the union. But by 1929 Walsh had lost his presidency and began a political swing to the right, eventually becoming a member of the New Guard in the early 1930s. Adela had moved even further right, establishing the Australian Women's Guild of Empire, a middle-class movement aimed at re-educating working-class women and dissuading them from industrial action. This change of political loyalties would have puzzled many of Pakie's patrons and it infuriated William Miles, who made Adela, his previous co-campaigner, the target of some vicious public ridicule. What neither Bee nor her father could have known was the way their lives would intersect with Adela's a decade on from that night in 1929, in the upstairs rooms of 219 Elizabeth Street, when Bernard Hesling, with Bee as his guide, finally landed on the sea coast of Bohemia.

Having installed Bernard safely into Pakie's care, Bee went to Brisbane for three days and on her return immediately sought him out. They had an intimate dinner in Pakie's private alcove, where other patrons' feet could be seen protruding under the curtains, but the potential romance never quite eventuated. Instead, they became friends and moved into opposite rooms in a large terrace house in Victoria Street in Darlinghurst, consisting of fourteen rooms. Bernard and Bee had attic rooms on the top floor. There were shared bathrooms and a single telephone guarded by the landlady who would sound a gong to announce an incoming call.

For many writers and artists who were employed in the city, or who made a living through freelance work, Darlinghurst was an ideal location. It offered a variety of accommodation choices through the gradual rise of flats and the breaking up of former mansions into inexpensive rooms, which provided a congenial mixture of freedom and affordable living. For Bee it was an area synonymous with unfettered cosmopolitanism. She wrote lovingly of: 'Sunday mornings in Victoria Street, Darlinghurst, Sydney, when I would stand on the roof outside my attic and listen to the bells of St Mary's Cathedral booming and swinging with the wind across Woolloomooloo Valley.'[21] Aspiring actors like Peter Finch and John 'Chips' Goffage, who would achieve fame as Chips Rafferty, whom Bee would come to know in the following decade, poets like Mary Gilmore and Kenneth Slessor and writers like Dulcie Deamer were long-term residents of Darlinghurst at various times. Deamer lived in Victoria Street at the same time as Bee. Perched in his apartment on the 'Alps' of Darlinghurst, Slessor's poetic gaze celebrated the area's mixture of charm and squalor in a series of poems and prose pieces. It was a chaotic blend of pedestrians, cars, taxis, trams and horses. Revellers in rumpled evening dress shared the pavement with early morning shoppers; neon light replaced the stars; and ships moored at Woolloomooloo Bay were visible from William Street. This gateway to upper Darlinghurst had been envisioned as a grand boulevard winding its way up the hill by various city planners in the nineteenth century but had fallen into decay, its derelict buildings home to impoverished artists like the Lindsay brothers, its seedy pubs haunted by Christopher Brennan in his days of decline. There were cheap eating establishments where a week's worth of meals could be purchased in advance for a pound. Pawn shops serviced the changing fortunes of residents and were often frequented by Bee, with copies of Shakespeare and Chaucer under her arm, declaring loudly to the startled proprietor that 'there is no God'.[22]

By comparison, her room up the hill in Victoria Street was large and fairly comfortable. She never cooked, living instead on oysters and ginger beer, though she was constantly brewing tea on the room's solitary gas ring.[23]

The 1920s, perhaps more than any other decade in the first half of the century, celebrated the visual aspects of modernity. The flappers' short skirts and cropped hair were designed for spectacle. Buildings climbed higher and the enormous span of the Harbour Bridge, as it edged towards completion, seemed to dwarf the city. The annual Artists' Ball attracted huge numbers of guests who competed for the most spectacular costume, including Dulcie Deamer, who wore her famous leopard-skin outfit, to a mixture of scandal and applause. For some bohemians, even everyday wardrobe choices had a political dimension. George Finey, by then a successful cartoonist and caricaturist, always dressed in tennis whites and never wore socks, as a way of expressing his opposition to capitalism. Geoffrey Cumine, poet and freelancer, wore green jackets and brass earrings and had the words 'To Let' tattooed across his forehead. Jack Lindsay affected a deliberate shabbiness to symbolise his rejection of bourgeois standards. But it was Bee's wardrobe choices—short, pleated skirts with men's flat patent leather shoes, or white shorts—that had begun to attract the attention of the newspapers, where her outfits were described in minute detail: 'Bee Miles has reappeared in Sydney again. I saw her last week alighting from a moving tram in Bent Street . . . her usual picturesque appearance accentuated by black pantaloons, golf socks . . . with her close Eton crop and inevitable cigarette she attracted a great deal of attention, people often wondering whether she is a girl or boy.'[24]

This was also the decade that saw the birth of the house—or more often, the flat—party.[25] The house party served an important role in an age where access to alcohol (and to women) was far more tightly controlled. The Lindsay brothers, Jack, Ray and Phil, along with George Finey, all described memorable parties where alcohol was consumed in vast amounts and outrageous behaviour was both expected and encouraged. It was also an opportunity for women to enjoy a more central role in bohemian culture, since they were excluded from the world of pubs, so intrinsic to male bohemian writers and artists. Even so, they remained largely background figures in most memoirs and recollections. Bee liked parties and being at the centre of activities. What she didn't like was the excessive consumption of alcohol. She was, like her father, largely temperate. This was despite the fact that William had inherited one the finest wine cellars in Sydney when his father died. It wasn't that she disapproved of alcohol, but it was more the fact that it made the conversation dull. For Bee, good conversation was an art form in itself:

> Nothing bores me more than going to a party where the company does nothing but drink. If drinking makes it truly gayer and more brilliantly conversational and forgetful of its priggeries and not merely dirty then the party is lovely: but as a rule it doesn't know when to stop and ends up a maudlin mess of unintelligibility.[26]

This may have been another reason that Bee felt so comfortable at Pakie's, which as noted, did not serve alcohol (though patrons often hid bottles amongst the pot plants). When she did attend parties, she found other ways to amuse herself, as one former bohemian recalled:

> She wasn't a brilliant talker but she wasn't a bad talker either. She had some good aphorisms, but she had lots of front and she had enough money of her own to get by on . . . I've seen her take a bath in the middle of a party and dry herself off in the lounge room, talking all the while. And I'm glad to say no one took much notice.[27]

Even though Bee was temperate in a movement that devoted much of its energy to procuring alcohol, on rare occasions she held her own parties. Hesling recalled one occasion when they were living in Darlinghurst. There was no alcohol, but Bee had ordered 'huge slab sandwiches' from the local ham-and-beef shop (the forerunner of the delicatessen). About thirty people turned up to find a note telling them to help themselves and that she would be back later. When she did return, she was dressed only in a swimming costume (illegal at the time) and with an extremely shy lifesaver called David, whom she literally hauled up the stairs. According to Hesling, she seemed surprised that a party was proceeding and bundled everyone out onto the landing apart from a highly embarrassed David, whom, she declared dramatically, had saved her life. Given Bee's outstanding ability as a swimmer, this is highly unlikely.

Along with the parties there were more organised and regular social gatherings, the most famous of which was the Noble Order of I Felici, Letterati, Conoscenti e Lunatici or Cheerful Lunatics. Its founder and 'Grand Master' was Sam Rosa. Rosa had an early career in radical socialist politics and connections with the IWW and, like Bee's father, was a polished stump orator. They would have known each other from mutual socialist circles. By 1925 he was working as an editor for the *Labour Daily* and, in his free time, presiding over the Noble Order meetings. Dulcie Deamer was one of its earliest members and became central to its proceedings. Deamer had forged a career as a freelancer in journalism and she also wrote a series of historical romances that enjoyed some success. Her chief claim to fame was as the Queen of Bohemia, having been officially crowned at one of the Noble Order meetings, where she had a central role in awarding kisses to male initiates. Other activities of the Order included organised games of mock athletics or battles, songs and performances—including Deamer's famous splits routine.[28] Its members were an eclectic group that included poets like Mary Gilmore (on rare occasions) and journalists like Eric Baume, as well as Bee. Saturday afternoon meetings at the Roma Café in Pitt Street were long and noisy and continued into the evening, when members moved on to other venues or to parties.

It's unknown how frequently Bee attended meetings, but she would have certainly been attracted to groups that challenged conventions and social mores, particularly those around sexuality.

Sexual activity was an important aspect of bohemian life and its rejection of conventional standards. Bee, who had been questioning the whole notion of sexual propriety from her teenage years, was, by her own admission, sexually active 'from the age of twenty-five'. This was also the age when she finally succeeded in escaping the asylum. However frank she was about her sexual exploits, she was always careful not to identify her conquests publicly. Privately, she kept meticulous records in case she became pregnant, something that may have occurred at some time during the 1920s:

> You hear a lot of talk about what a wild girl Bee used to be.
> A lot of it was Bee's fault. She wasn't a bad girl, but she liked
> to shock people. I've heard her come into the Angel Hotel
> and say in a loud voice 'Just been down to Melbourne for my
> abortion'. Of course she'd done no such thing![29]

Despite these protestations (discreetly described by Souter in his 1956 portrait of Bee, as being by 'a former suitor'), it is entirely plausible that Bee could have had an abortion. Contraception was difficult to obtain and she was adamant that she never wanted children 'because she wasn't worth reproducing'. But she was also a strong believer in sexual freedom and thought that the practice of infanticide was extremely rational. Hesling once said he never knew of 'any man who slept with her who remained with her. I also don't remember any man who fought to see more of her.'[30]

Hesling's cryptic comment might relate to an anecdote about Bee when she was living in Darlinghurst at the height of the Golden Decade. She had embarked on a relationship with a man, whose identity, yet again, is unknown. While his ardour had cooled, Bee's had not. She wanted to continue their affair. In a mark of desperation, he confided to some friends that he had booked a passage on a ship departing that evening, because he had to 'get away from that woman'. Unfortunately, Bee learned about his intended escape and bolted down to the harbour as the ship was leaving. Much to the horror of her departing lover, she is said to have leapt up, taken hold of the anchor rope, and swung back and forth across the bow of the ship, trying to land on the deck. It is impossible to know how true this story is, but it's highly plausible given Bee's propensity for risk, her compulsiveness and her determination to get her own way.

Even though Bee is often remembered in historical portraits and memoirs of the bohemian period, she was not a central figure and like other female bohemians, her literary aspirations were rarely if ever mentioned, subsumed by a focus on her appearance and behaviour. She seems to have moved in and out of various groups and clubs, failing or not choosing to develop significant friendships apart from her relationships with Bernard Hesling, Pakie and the communist writer Phyllis Ophel. Or perhaps it was not her choice to make. Some bohemians became legendary casualties of the life they embraced, like Joe Lynch,[31] the subject of Slessor's poem 'Five Bells', and Anna Brennan, the daughter of Christopher Brennan, whose short but mercurial life has been well documented. For a select few the opposite happened, and they moved from the periphery to the centre of mainstream artistic culture. Others simply returned to the middle-class lives they had rejected and in turn rejected their old associations, including Bee. Some, like a former boyfriend, who became the manager of a prominent bookstore in the city, gave her firm instructions not to enter his store. Others when they saw Bee avoided her because she had started to push the bohemian penchant for outrageous behaviour beyond the limits of safety: 'People think I'm dangerous or something like that. I'm lonely. They don't want to be seen out with me so I have to be self sufficient.'[32]

Jack Lindsay described the intellectual and cultural milieu of the 'roaring twenties' as a rejection of authority in the aftermath of the First World War and a fear that they were living in the shadow of another, pending catastrophe. Dulcie Deamer saw the same period as an expression of a post-war *joie de vivre* and a sense that everything from now on was going to be 'good oh'. These central figures in bohemian Sydney represented its two philosophical bookends. Lindsay's interest in the aesthetics of a new vision for Australian artistic expression was almost diametrically opposed to Deamer's anti-intellectual pursuit of fun and spectacle, but in other ways they were not so different. Both were attracted to nonconformity and libertarian ideals and each in their own way cultivated a provocative stance towards what they considered the prosaic nature of mainstream Australian social values. They were Bee's contemporaries and, although she never identified them, it is clear they had an influence in shaping her ideas.[33]

The bohemian values Bee held were not a temporary fashion or an expression of youthful rebellion. A rejection of bourgeois propriety; an adherence to the notion of the artist–genius and the centrality of individualism; the embrace of modern technology, urban living and the carnivalesque nature of life—all were elements of bohemianism she understood and responded to. She was not interested in any kind of vertical ascension, and she had neither the desire nor the impetus to change. Looking back on the Golden Decade thirty years on, she wrote: 'True bohemians place no value on clothes, on social position nor on money, provided they are not forced to live in abject poverty. There is only one true Bohemian in Sydney.'[34]

At the end of the decade, whether she chose to recognise it or not, change was coming. The New York stock market crash of 1929 heralded a worldwide economic collapse. The genteel poverty experienced by many bohemians was dwarfed in the face of devastating financial hardship across the country, with one in three Australian men unemployed. The Golden Decade was over, and the Great Depression had begun.

7

Playing the Game

'I hated the smug respectability of suburban life and the coldly
polite reproofs of the people who thought me too much.'

Bee Miles, *Arrow*, 1 January 1932

The Cenotaph sits in Martin Place, one of Sydney's busiest
thoroughfares. Its centrepiece is an austere granite block, carved
in the shape of an altar stone. A single stone wreath decorates its
surface, while two bronze figures guard its flanks—a soldier to the
east and a sailor to the west. In 1929 they stood as sombre witnesses
before the streams of shoppers and office workers who passed before
them: silent reminders of the cloud that had enveloped the world a
decade before. As the crowds hurried by, many thought about the
loved ones they had lost fighting in far-off countries, or the husbands
and fathers who had returned wounded in body or mind or both.
Of the 331,781 men who had enlisted to fight overseas during the
war, more than 65 per cent had become casualties. Everyone knew
someone . . . To the right of the Cenotaph stood the GPO, where so
many of these men had signed up to fight. To its left, Challis House
and the well-appointed offices of William Miles, who had waged his
own long and bitter campaign against the conscription of Australians
to fight on foreign soil. He had won that battle but the victory had

been quickly overshadowed by the legend of the Anzacs and the near religious reverence of their sacrifice. So great was the public need for commemoration that the premier, Jack Lang, was persuaded to set aside £10,000 for the memorial's construction, even though he, like William Miles, had opposed conscription during the war. On 21 February 1929, the Cenotaph was unveiled by the new premier, Thomas Bavin. Sir John Monash, famous war hero, gave the speech.

Eleven months later, in early January 1930, the passing public was witness to another, less edifying spectacle. A young woman was perched on the side of the Cenotaph smoking a cigarette. When Constable Masters asked her to move on, she refused. 'The Cenotaph,' she said, 'is not a sacred place; no dead bodies are interred there and no sermons are preached there.'[1] Constable Masters disagreed. He found her behaviour 'offensive' to him and arrested her. The magistrate at Central Police Court agreed as well and fined her £1. She chose to serve seven days in gaol instead and was sent to the State Reformatory for Women at Long Bay on the edges of the city. After news of the arrest spread, an unidentified person came forward to pay her fine, only to find that someone else paid it earlier. She was released after spending just one night of her sentence. It wasn't her first arrest, but it was her first experience of prison, an event that sparked the media interest that would continue for many years to come.[2]

———

Much of Bee's early rebellion during her school years had been a reaction to the First World War. Her political views had been formed through her rejection of its validity—a rejection that had seen her isolated from her fellow students and teachers. She had witnessed police raids on her home because of her father's political activities and saw her family ostracised by the local community. At home, despite supporting her father's politics, she challenged his authority and the harshness of his punishments. As a result, he rejected her and consigned her to three-and-a-half years of involuntary restraint.

Within the asylums, her life had been turned upside down and her personal freedom taken away. Every movement was monitored and controlled in pursuit of the elusive 'cure'. Every response she made was measured against a set of standards that she increasingly came to reject. She neither forgave nor forgot the three agents of the state that had been instrumental in her committal: the police, the judiciary and the medical profession. The 'conventional authority' they represented had deprived her of her freedom and plunged her life into chaos. Now she began to reject this authority at every opportunity. What she wanted was freedom of movement, but her choice of movement meant transgression. Being young and female only compounded the problem. Still bitter about her arrest, she observed: 'People in London sit on the pedestal of Nelson's monument. Children in Washington sit in the lap of Abe Lincoln's statue but girls in Sydney must not sit on the Cenotaph.'[3]

Bee's feelings towards her father were more ambivalent. He had been the main protagonist in her confinement and banishment from the family. The fact that she had deliberately chosen the Cenotaph as the location for her first public act of political dissent was no accident, and could have been a gesture of support for her father's wartime resistance. Equally, it might have been a way of embarrassing him, with her arrest in full view of his offices. It could easily have been both, but in any case her father's response is unrecorded. The rebellious behaviour Bee had honed during her periods of committal was sharpened by her exposure to bohemian culture and its celebration of the carnivalesque nature of human existence. Social conventions that were in the way of pursuing pleasure and living life as an art form were to be challenged or ignored. Speed, movement, freedom, risk and spectacle—and the irresistible lure of machines—all converged to produce what she called the 'game': 'Just that; a favourite way of having fun on my own. One day shall write a paper on the Art, Fine Points and Ethics of this game. To play it one only needs a little agility and a little courage.'[4]

It had begun with cars, leaping on to the back or sideboards—a sight that both astonished and amused those who witnessed it, like the young Bernard Hesling. At the start, even the police seemed to tolerate it. Bee was allowed to join the welcome parade for the famous female pilot Amy Johnson, when she arrived in Sydney after her epic flight from England to Australia in 1930.[5] Bee perched in the spare tyre cavity of Johnson's car all the way from Mascot Airport to Darlinghurst. And when a crowd of 2000 marched from Railway Square to the Domain on the anniversary of the Russian Revolution in 1931, Bee was pulled on her bicycle by an obliging police car. Newspapers reports, which initially ran under headings such as 'Strange girl's antics', began to be more personalised. She was the 'Bumper Bar Beauty' or the 'Bumper Bar Girl'; the 'bare-headed, bare-legged girl', whose poor mind had been overturned by too much study. She was considered harmless and her appearance brightened up an 'otherwise dull city'.[6]

But it wasn't entirely harmless. Twelve months after her triumphant ride on Johnson's car, Bee was involved in a serious accident in the city. She was thrown from the luggage carrier of a car that had braked suddenly in traffic. She was taken to hospital and treated for a fractured ankle. Shortly after that she began to use a bicycle, but she never really cycled. Instead, she used it to move closer to cars and trams, where she would take hold from behind and be pulled along. This increased her speed but also the danger, though not always from other vehicles. In December 1931, newspapers reported that Bee had been attempting to take hold of a tram turning into William Street when she was pulled off her bicycle by a policeman. The wind had blown 'the inevitable' cigarette she had been smoking into her knapsack and set it alight. Once the policeman extinguished the flames, she got back on the bike and resumed her journey.[7] Three months later, she was hit from behind by a car. Although the bicycle was damaged, she escaped injury. The driver of the car wasn't so lucky. On seeing the damage, Bee became 'frightfully angry' and punched him in the face. After pleading guilty 'under intense provocation', she was given a good behaviour bond.[8]

By now stories about Bee were appearing in the newspapers on a weekly basis. She was frequently included in round-ups of news-worthy events in the city and sometimes further afield. Towards the end of 1931 a story was circulating that Bee had 'held up' a train at Guyra in the New England region of New South Wales. After the car she had been travelling in broke down near a railway line, Bee stepped onto the tracks and waved down an oncoming train. The driver, most likely in a state of shock, stopped and she casually climbed on board and proceeded to the next town, where she arranged for a car to return and tow the broken-down vehicle. She was fined an unspecified amount.[9]

Perhaps as a way of shaping her growing public image Bee gave a lengthy interview to the *Arrow*, which appeared on New Year's Day 1932. Given that the holidays were a notoriously quiet period for newspaper copy, the *Arrow* gave her a double-page spread under the headline 'The Terror of the Bumper Bar'. Carefully dressed in a tight-fitting black dress and black silk stockings, Bee constructed a profile of herself that was designed to be both benign and shocking. Gliding over the history of her early life, her difficulties conforming to Abbotsleigh's regulations and her family's 'tiring' of her eccentricities, she 'found' herself in an asylum where she witnessed some inhumane practices and was seduced by a female nurse. She spoke of being in prison and her supposed breakdown at university from 'over study', claiming she left because she was bored. Her one ambition, she said, was to be 'a really serious writer'. Then she turned to the topic of relationships. She had been in love 'five times' she said but this time, with her current 'sweetheart', it was different. He was an intellectual and able to converse on her favourite topics: psychology, literature and history. But he was also broke and was leaving that afternoon to find work interstate. She might follow him or she might not. This brought her on to the subject of marriage. There was nothing to be gained from marriage—in fact it was tyranny.

It ends freedom for women and when freedom is taken away 'love dies'. Women who want to have babies should be able to do so without stigma, whether they are married or not, like they could in the Soviet Union. After all, why should some priest 'chanting a few words over them' make a difference? 'What has the church go to do with nature?' she asked. Knowing the article would cause controversy, she finished the interview with a rhetorical question: 'I suppose you must think it terrible that a person my age should be wild like this?'[10]

The public response is unrecorded but the experience set a trend for Bee. When her repeated attempts to have her manuscripts published failed, she began to circulate selections from them in newspapers. It also whetted her appetite for public commentary. In the 1930s, along with her ambition to be a published writer, she still harboured a desire to be a critic. 'Critics,' she told a Brisbane reporter in 1929, 'have brains, mould public opinion and set standards.'[11] Providing formal interviews was her way of controlling the narrative—something that was becoming increasingly difficult.

Three weeks after the *Arrow* interview Bee's grandmother died. She was ninety years old. Obituaries paid tribute to her remarkable voice, her contribution to both sacred and secular music and her many works of charity. According to her wishes, she was buried with the songs that had been written for her during her successful career, along with the nineteenth century romantic novel *Wanda*.[12] There was no religious service. Bee had lost the one constant in her family and her refuge.

———

Bee's crowning act of 1932 coincided with one of the most seminal moments in the city's history, the opening of the Sydney Harbour Bridge. The idea of constructing a bridge to link the northern shore of the harbour with the city had been in existence since colonial times, but actual planning did not commence until 1914, only to be interrupted by the onset of the First World War. Finally, in 1923, a ceremony was held to mark the beginning of construction. Throughout the 1920s Sydneysiders watched the slow progression of the giant steel arch's two sides inching towards each other, as the bridge's span rose to its final height of 134 metres above the sea. Despite the stock market crash of 1929 and the crippling financial Depression that followed, construction of the bridge continued, providing desperately needed employment for some 1600 men. The project was overseen by John Bradfield, who also supervised the building of the Cenotaph, using the same granite to decorate the bridge's concrete pylons.

It is estimated that around a million people converged on Sydney on 19 March 1932 to witness the bridge's official opening. At the time the city's entire population was only 1,256,000. People had travelled from everywhere and took up every available public space to witness the spectacle. Parks and streets were crammed and overflowing, while the more agile perched on every available fence and rooftop. Trams were literally stopped in their tracks, unable to move safely through the swarming crowds. Macquarie Street was ablaze with colour as floral decorations marked the solemn progress of the governor's escort down to the bridge entry for the official opening.

It had been assumed that the governor, Sir Philip Game, would open the bridge, but Premier Lang, in defiance of protocol and imperial rank, had decided to award himself the honour. Lang, by then a figure of so much controversy, was seen by conservative forces as the harbinger of a Bolshevik revolution and unforgivingly disloyal to Britain. In a climate where the division between Left and Right politics was growing increasingly violent, Lang used his official speech to describe the bridge as a unifying symbol for Australia's future. But before the premier had a chance to cut the official ribbon, Francis De Groot, a member of the extreme right-wing paramilitary group the New Guard, charged forward and sliced it with his sword 'in the name of the decent and respectable people of New South Wales'. De Groot was quickly pulled from his horse by

Superintendent William MacKay and taken away to Darlinghurst Reception House for examination. In the meantime, the ribbon was hastily put together again so the premier could cut it and the bridge was opened. As the cannons fired below and planes flew overhead, marching bands and processions of decorated floats paraded past the crowds, while underneath, the harbour's waters were brimming with ships, ferries and smaller craft, crammed with waving passengers. Then hundreds of thousands of people rushed forth to march across the bridge for the first time. Three people died, another 500 fainted and 300 children were lost in the crush. Next came the vehicles, and perched on the bonnet of the first truck to cross the bridge was a slim, lithe and triumphant Bee Miles.[13]

After being observed at the Reception House for 24 hours, De Groot was declared sane. He was found guilty of offensive behaviour and fined £5. He later sued Superintendent MacKay for wrongful arrest and was awarded an undisclosed settlement.[14] One of his many supporters later sent him a cigarette case with the words 'he is not insane' engraved across its width.

There were no reported arrests for Bee on that day or for the remainder of 1932. She may have used this time to finish her first manuscript 'Advance Australia Fair', her first-person account of her committals and escapes from hospital, and to focus on the relationship she spoke about in her *Arrow* interview. She had fallen, she later said, 'heavily in love for the first time'. Although this man has sometimes been identified incorrectly as Brian Harper, his true identity remains unknown.[15] Bee identified him only by the letter 'P' and said he was a 'businessman'.

———

From the time she took up residence in Darlinghurst in the late 1920s Bee had stayed in and around Sydney, apart from the occasional brief trip to Brisbane where she had relations on her mother's side. In 1933 she suddenly decided to relocate to Melbourne.

The reasons are unclear. As a city, Melbourne was more conservative than Sydney, and the last time she had been there had not been a positive experience. It was during one of her escapes from Gladesville Mental Hospital and, as discussed earlier, she was arrested at a boarding house, placed under observation and then escorted back to Sydney where her punishment was severe.

But by April Bee was again staying in a Melbourne boarding house. She had taken up residence at Osborne House in Nicholson Street, Fitzroy. Bee described the proprietor, Mrs Inez Meagher, as 'a bright soul', whom she admired intensely for her 'defence of those in trouble' and, importantly for Bee, her philosophy of non-interference.[16] Mrs Meagher also won her approval for being a Christian Scientist. In a rare moment of praise for religion, Bee approved of Christian Scientists because they rejected medical intervention. She felt secure at Osborne House, and perhaps Inez reminded her of Pakie. She certainly felt confident that Inez 'wouldn't give her away' and that Osborne House would make an 'excellent hide out'. Within a matter of weeks, she was in need of one. She had come to the attention of the Melbourne newspaper reporters. Mistakenly identified as a 'pert Melbourne girl', she was described as an 'astounding sight' in the 'staid decorum' of the St Kilda Police Court, where her brief skirt 'revealed her knees'. She was charged with riding a bicycle in a negligent manner, having been seen being towed by a vehicle at a speed of 30 miles per hour (just under 50 kilometres per hour). When asked why she had a policeman's whistle around her neck, Bee told the magistrate it was to make people move out of the way as they didn't always hear the bell and she happily gave a demonstration. While the journalists present were amused, the magistrate wasn't. He knew he had seen her before but couldn't quite recall the circumstance. Bee tried unsuccessfully to negotiate a lighter penalty with the magistrate, claiming she couldn't afford to pay and would have to do the time instead. She didn't help her case by telling him he was horrible. The magistrate remained unimpressed and fined her £2, in lieu of which she spent seven days in gaol.[17] A week in gaol seems like a rather severe punishment for such a minor offense. Boys on bicycles hanging onto the back of trams were a common sight in cities across Australia. Stockingless, smoking young women doing the same thing were not.

Less than two weeks later, and only recently released from the Women's Prison, she was engaged in a 'spirited exchange' with three magistrates at a South Melbourne Court. The hearing was for a similar offence that had occurred earlier on 4 April. This may have been the incident the St Kilda Court magistrate was trying to remember. Initially, Bee was compliant, assuring the court that a fine would be a deterrent and that she had already sent the bicycle back to the shop and had given up cycling. While the magistrates were deliberating, she approached the bench and asked one of them to 'put in a good word' for her. It seemed to work. The case was adjourned for three months on the condition she did not cause any more trouble on a bicycle, otherwise the punishment would be severe. 'How severe?' Bee inquired. But by now the magistrate had lost patience and told her to be quiet and not make 'an even bigger fool of herself'. Obviously feeling relaxed at the reprieve she had just received, Bee returned volley: 'Don't speak to me like that. It is contempt of court to insult a prisoner.' The journalists loved this performance and their reports were reprinted in Adelaide and Perth.

Despite the magistrates' warnings and the increasing police attention, Bee continued to indulge in 'the game' at every opportunity. One day in town she spotted 'a gorgeous car come rolling gently down the street'. She jumped on the back but someone alerted the chauffeur, who stopped and pointed her out to a policeman as she walked away. Several days later she was strolling down St Kilda Road when a policeman stopped her and asked for her name. 'You see,' he said seriously, 'the other day you were riding on the Lord Mayor's car and that's not the thing to do is it?' Bee was delighted.[18] On one occasion she was spotted on her bicycle by two policemen who ordered her to stop. She refused and fled into a nearby park with the police following on foot. Pedalling furiously, she led them around trees and flowerbeds and down garden paths. In desperation, one of the police commandeered a bicycle from a passing citizen and the chase continued. Finally, she was caught when another policeman appeared on a motorcycle and blocked her path. She described the experience as 'joy'.[19] By now she was starting to gain a reputation with the tram drivers as well. She claimed that they were putting sand on the tracks so it would blow in her eyes when she was approaching them from the rear. All trams carried a quantity of sand under the driver's compartment, which would be released when the tracks were oily. In retaliation she started a campaign of ringing the tram bell after the tram had stopped. This infuriated the drivers and again brought the attention of the police.

One busy Saturday morning in Bourke Street in the middle of the city she was spotted ringing the bell of a tram. The police ordered her to get down, to which she responded that she was doing no harm. Eventually she left the tram but immediately tried to board a passing car. After being refused by four different drivers and with the police in hot pursuit, she jumped on the back of a vehicle as it pulled away and disappeared triumphantly up Swanston Street. She was soon in court again. Facing yet another magistrate, Bee acknowledged that the evidence given by two constables was accurate but denied that her behaviour was offensive. 'I wasn't doing any harm to any member of the public. Nobody complained but you,' she told the police witness. After the prosecutor read out her previous convictions, she turned to the crowded court and exclaimed, 'Dash it all, men, the city should be glad to have such a carefree citizen to brighten up an otherwise dull city,' which sounded suspiciously like she was quoting from earlier newspaper articles. 'Will you keep away from the city?' the prosecutor asked, trying a different approach. 'No,' Bee responded firmly. 'Why should I? Just wink your other eye and leave me alone.' By now the gallery, the police witnesses, court reporters and even the Bench began to laugh. Under further questioning Bee told the court that she'd been arrested in Sydney and admitted to psychiatric hospitals. Perhaps realising that she had said too much, she approached the Bench and asked the magistrate to be 'a sport'. In a mark of seeming desperation, the magistrate asked her if she would promise to stop the offending. 'I never make promises,' she responded, sealing her fate.[20] It wasn't the outcome she'd hoped for but in that moment she began to understand the power of performance and the way she could capture the attention of court. She was remanded for medical observation to Mont Park Reception House, where she was diagnosed as 'hypo maniacal'.[21] After seven days she was extradited back to Sydney. The experience had been fun, she reflected, and 'tremendous sport, but the cops were tough!'[22]

For the citizens of Melbourne, it had been enough.

———

For someone who held the medical profession in contempt, Bee had a fascination with hospitals. She had qualified for medicine when she gained entry to Sydney University and had seriously contemplated it as a career choice, before enrolling in an arts degree. Her experiences in psychiatric hospitals had convinced her that the majority of male doctors were disingenuous, and used their profession and the deference it awarded them to increase their social status and access to women. But she liked hospitals and, in particular, anaesthetics. Sometime in the early 1930s she underwent an elaborate process to fake an attack of tonsillitis in order to procure an operation. By 1934 she claimed to have had fifteen general anaesthetics and admitted she had trouble resisting the smell of ether. Because of its proximity, Sydney Hospital in Macquarie Street became her regular haunt. She had even had a voluntary job there in the late 1920s, sterilising bandages, but was purportedly driven out by the nursing association. By 1933 her presence at the hospital was becoming a nuisance. Eschewing her own doctrine of 'non-interference', she had started examining patients and attempting to remove their dressings. The more the medical staff ejected her, the more she returned. When a clearly exasperated Dr Harris wrote to the medical superintendent at the Darlinghurst Reception House on 26 August 1933, he said that her visits over the previous 48 hours had been 'intolerably frequent'. She was escorted to the Reception House by the police.

At the Reception House she gave her address as 14 Roslyn Gardens, Darlinghurst. Under examination her physical condition was described as good, although she had bruises on her arms and legs. Her weight was around 66 kilograms; she'd gained 12 and a half kilograms since her first visit to the Reception House in 1923. Over the next two days she was further examined by doctors. They described her as 'boisterous and excitable . . . impulsive . . . lacking control'. She refused to admit that her conduct was 'extraordinary'. Most concerning was the fact that she was 'unable to restrain herself from behaviour unfitting to a woman of her years and education, such as jumping onto trams, riding on the backs of motor cars and chuckling policemen under the chin'.[23] She was a nuisance to the police and caused confusion in the streets for motorists. Unlike De Groot, who was released from the Reception House after 24 hours, Bee was detained for six days and then escorted to Kenmore Mental Hospital in Goulburn, back under the care of the superintendent Dr Gordon Moffitt. No one sent her a cigarette case.

Attempting to remove the dressings from patients was indeed strange behaviour and a marked departure from Bee's usual forms of disruption, which were always staged in public and focused on movement. While she often discussed and dissected 'the game', analysing both its purpose and the reactions it evoked, she never mentioned interfering with patients' bandages or provided any explanation for her behaviour.

Bee was still in a manic state when she arrived at Kenmore. She was pacing back and forth, refusing to sit down and smoking constantly, yet she appeared to recover quickly. By the end of two weeks, she was doing jigsaw puzzles and getting on well with the nursing staff. But she was still refusing to acknowledge that her behaviour was somehow 'extraordinary' or wrong and insisted that she rode on the back of cars because 'she had guts. Other girls have not the guts though they would love to do it if they dared'. By October she was writing six letters a day, including letters to 'two young men' about writing a book. She started to insist that she be allowed out. Surprisingly Dr Moffitt agreed. In fact, he had already been writing to her father on the same topic.

The last time Bee had been in Kenmore under Moffitt's care, he had provided a statement to her father's lawyer confirming that she was 'insane and required to be kept in order like a child'. Now, two weeks into her stay, he wrote to William stating that Bee was 'not very bad mentally and is well in bodily health'. Might she be able to be discharged to a willing relative, he asked. He thought that William could appreciate the difficulty of the hospital's position. William didn't, and he sent a curt response the next day stating that his daughter was 'quite capable of looking after herself *to her own satisfaction.* (Beyond that I hold no particular opinion)'. Undeterred, three weeks later Moffitt wrote to William again. This time he had a possible solution. Bee had written to her cousin Gordon Mitchell, a distant relative of her grandmother, and he was willing to assume responsibility for her supervision. Would William agree to his daughter being released into Mitchell's care, he wrote, adding that 'she had been very good'. William was becoming impatient. He wrote back by courier, stating he had 'no control whatever' over his daughter. His only influence was the weekly allowance, which he refused to pay when she was in gaol or in hospital. Again, he repeated his statement that she was quite capable of looking after herself 'to her own satisfaction'. Gordon Mitchell, on the other hand, took a different approach. In his formal request to have Bee released into his care, he claimed to be one of 'the few people who had a certain amount of control over her'. She listened to him and took his advice. If Dr Moffitt agreed, he would call for Bee and drive her immediately to his mother's house in Harrow Road, Kogarah, a southern Sydney suburb. Somewhat bravely, given Bee's history, he agreed to take on 'the full responsibility of her future behaviour'. Moffitt leapt at the chance and told Mitchell he 'could come for her at any time', adding, 'I need hardly say that we are not anxious to keep her here.' On 25 October Bee left the hospital with her cousin. She was granted a leave of absence for twelve months on the condition she returned at the end of October 1934 for examination.[24]

When October came, and following an inquiry from the hospital, a rather embarrassed Gordon Mitchell wrote to Moffitt admitting that he didn't know where Bee was. She had gone back to Melbourne to join in the city's centenary celebrations and he had no way of contacting her. He did add that her mental condition was the best it had been in years and that she was listening to his advice, which was, he wrote, something new. Even though she was missing in action, Bee was granted a further period of leave for twelve months, provided she remained in Mitchell's care and that she presented for examination every three months. It's unlikely that she attended or that she was in Melbourne for the centenary. Whether she listened to her cousin's advice as he claimed is a moot point. She was determined to keep challenging 'conventional authority' by playing the game:

> I have been told that I show poorness of judgement because
> I continue my wild ways though I've been jailed and mental
> hospitalised for 'em many times. But I consider that hanging
> on to trams and cars with my bike is the safest for me, at
> least, to ride and that riding bumper-bars and mudguards is
> a thoroughly innocent way of having fun. If I capitulate it
> simply gives encouragement to the police to make further
> restricting laws. So I refuse to capitulate.[25]

8

Jumping the Rattler

'Ladies and gentlemen are persons of great moral courage who do, say, eat, dress, as know whom and use what language they please, without asking anybody's approval or permission. I am not always trying to prove myself a lady. I was born one and I'm damned if I care what people think of me.'

Bee Miles, 'Dictionary by a Bitch', p. 11

Superintendent William MacKay was not a man to be trifled with. The son of a Glaswegian policeman, he immigrated to Sydney in 1910 and joined the local police force. His knowledge of shorthand allowed him to compile detailed reports of anti-conscription speeches at Domain during the First World War, leading to the successful prosecution of many of William Miles' co-campaigners. MacKay came to prominence during the infamous razor gang wars of the 1920s and was credited with bringing an end to the gangs' vicious attacks. His rise through the ranks was accelerated by his hardline approach to striking miners at Rothbury near Newcastle, where a young miner was shot by the police and up to 50 others wounded. By the 1930s he was directing the members of his force to infiltrate the growing membership of the paramilitary New Guard as well as the Communist Party. His reputation was cemented when he pulled a sword-wielding De Groot off his horse in front of the crowds and dignitaries on that fateful day on the Harbour Bridge, captured on camera for all the country to see.[1] Somewhat curiously for an officer of such rank and status, Bee claimed that he had made time to hold a meeting with her, where a verbal agreement was reached. She would be given a three-year period of grace from arrests but after that, if she failed to be 'normal' and 'settle down', she would face the consequences from the members of his force. By 1934 the period of grace, if it had existed, was up, or else MacKay had rescinded the offer.[2] Bee had a long list of outstanding warrants or 'blues' and was technically still a patient at Kenmore. Suddenly Sydney, which had always been her refuge, was closing in on her. She was, she admitted, tired of going to gaol. If she returned to Melbourne, she would undoubtedly suffer a worse fate and end up in a Reception House, only to be sent back to Kenmore. Instead, she turned her attention northwards, embarking on a six-month trek across the country, recording her experiences along the way. Her travel diaries would form the basis for her second manuscript, which she called 'I Leave in a Hurry', a picaresque account of her epic journey through nearly every jurisdiction in Australia.

Travel writing in the early twentieth century was predominantly a male profession, though there were notable exceptions like the journalist Ernestine Hill, whose research and travel to produce *The Great Australian Loneliness* overlapped at times with Bee's journey. Other female writers like Kylie Tennant and Jean Devanny travelled and wrote from political and ideological motivation. The remarkable Eve Langley, whose life mirrors Bee's experiences in several ways, journeyed to reclaim her beloved Gippsland, rendered so vividly in *The Pea-Pickers*. In the 1930s, when access to rural and remote Australia was limited and expensive, travel writing was popular and, when successful, highly lucrative—with sales exceeding most other types of Australian writing.[3]

Regardless of motive or aspiration, women could not simply move around the country alone without a legitimate reason for travel. They risked being suspected of prostitution and a likely arrest for vagrancy if they did. A vagrancy charge was often preferred by police, as it resulted in a longer prison sentence. In New South Wales continued amendments to the *Police Offences Act*, the *Vagrancy Act* and the *Lunacy Act* increased police powers to regulate public order and exercise moral judgement on what constituted appropriate public behaviour. Hence, the familiar statement by individual police when they arrested Bee, that 'she was offensive to me'. Similar powers were extended to police in Victoria and South Australia. Even being in possession of money was not enough to avoid arrest under the *Vagrancy Act* and the onus was on the suspect to prove that their finances were obtained honestly.[4] Hesling recalled that when Bee was away, he often received calls from 'Woop Woop constabulary' in the middle of the night, to verify that she had a regular income from her father.[5] In the 1930s the rate of arrest for women charged with lunacy also rose substantially.[6]

Despite the risks, remaining in Sydney was now more dangerous, and in early April 1934 Bee 'packed a bag and cleared out'. She took the precaution of using a circuitous route out of the city to avoid the police at North Sydney, where she had more outstanding warrants. She persuaded a reluctant driver to allow her to ride on the mudguard of his car to Newcastle, more than 160 kilometres. From there she made her way slowly up the coast, obtaining lifts on motorbikes and trucks more easily than cars. Often the lifts were in delivery vans, including an unpleasant ride in a fish truck. Unlike the cities, where the abundance of vehicles enabled her to jump on without detection, on this trip she would have to resort to putting out her hand or approaching a vehicle to request a lift. The results were not always successful, and she had long periods of waiting between rides. Because the average man, she told herself, was 'afraid of strange women',[7] she must always present herself as a 'lady' to improve her chances of getting cars to stop. She had abandoned her customary shorts and bare legs and wore a conventional dress, stockings and shoes. It seemed to work:

> When I speak to the driver, saying 'going far?' in my polite way, he gazes hard at me, trying to sum me up. He forms a good opinion of me because I'm clean and neatly dressed. Most men judge women by their general appearance (largely by their clothes), first, last and always because they haven't sufficient judgement to see below the surface.[8]

This tactic would have also helped her to avoid arrest, at least in the early stages of her trip. (Eve Langley and her sister wore men's overalls on their travels in rural Victoria in the 1920s and were arrested for impersonating males.[9]) 'The more normal I am,' Bee noted ironically, 'the easier it is for me to be dishonest.'[10] But she did wear a large belt, called a cestus, which she had made in Sydney. It had a pocket on the inside and a harness buckle. There was a pouch suspended on two loops that contained her essentials: tobacco, hanky, pen and paper, and powder and rouge for 'luring purposes'.[11]

Bee's travels along the north coast were largely without incident and she was often given free accommodation at local hotels. Obliging drivers paid for her meals, while the proprietor of a local garage let her sleep in a room above his repair shop. Most drivers were male, and she was sometimes in the company of two or three men in a car, but often it was just Bee and the driver for long stretches in isolated country. Though she frequently had to rebuff their sexual overtures (businessmen she described as intent on business), she only recorded one incident where she was genuinely concerned at being alone with a driver, who began to act strangely. She contemplated throwing herself from the car but thought he might chase her through the bush. In her fear she began to 'sniffle'. Then the driver asked her if she was getting a cold. 'This question reassures me because no murderer would be so courteous as to enquire about the health of an intended victim. Sit calmly by his side now and do not tremble when the bush comes closer and bellbirds toll.'[12] Occasionally she met people she knew, like the commercial traveller who picked her up near Port Macquarie. The conversation was delicate, and Bee was discreet about the encounter, but added 'he tried to be very polite and kind because some years before he had got me into what might have been serious trouble.' The nature of the trouble was left unexplained.

Bee's other fear was being extradited at the Queensland border, though she passed through without incident. After stopping briefly in Brisbane and noting that the city's one redeeming feature was that patrons were allowed to smoke in cinemas, she headed north. She was writing all the time, chronicling the towns she passed through, adding brief descriptions of their main features and anchoring them to geographical locations, but rarely describing the scenery around her. She was far more interested in her interactions with people she met than the physical environment they inhabited. People's speech seemed to fascinate her, particularly the sounds and cadence of language, which she often compared to music. Bee loved the richness and humour of Australian vernacular, recording chance conversations verbatim, and adding footnotes to explain the meaning of local expressions and phrases, as well as the botanical names for local native plants. She was writing about Australia but aiming for an international audience. On rare occasions, she addressed her readers directly:

> Oh girls! Have achieved the hitherto impossible. For years
> have tried to persuade the drivers of petrol-wagons to allow
> me to ride beside them. But no! those cold, stern men of fuel
> have always refused. But now am sitting in a Plume wagon
> some miles from Caboolture. Am snugly tucked in with a
> handsome driver beside me. Will lay bets that no one else
> could do it. Am sheathed in vanity. Today's a red-letter day.[13]

Throughout the 1930s there was speculation about Bee's income. Initially, she had received an allowance of £8 a week. Along with the money her father provided, she received a small income from her grandmother, and while its amount and duration are unclear, payments would have ceased in 1932 when her grandmother died. There was no further provision for Bee in her will. Her main source of income was the £3 a week her father had agreed to pay her unless she was in gaol or an asylum. In 1933 the nominal male income was £4 1s 6d, but in reality many earned much less. Women's wages were 50 per cent of men's and frequent arbitration and union intervention limited women's access to full-time work. Most workers whose income was £1 or less were women.[14] Though Bee's income assured her a reasonable, if frugal, existence in the city, the distances she was covering on this journey meant she had to try to secure extra income or cut costs wherever she could. She was constantly worried about money and never stayed in hotels unless she was offered free accommodation, which was often the case, provided she did some housework in return. She earned a little money selling her stories to local newspapers in Maryborough and Bundaberg, which was some relief. As a single woman, she was not eligible for the limited entitlements available to white females during the 1930s, which were tied to marital status, children or old age. Unemployment benefits were not introduced until 1944. Being arrested for vagrancy, prostitution or lunacy was a constant source of anxiety.

Even so, Bee's situation was vastly better than many around her. At the height of the Great Depression, with the economy in total collapse, competition for the few jobs that existed was fierce. With one in three people unemployed, and many others on reduced hours, it is estimated that, in New South Wales alone, approximately 2000 families either left or were evicted from their homes and forced to live in unemployment camps or ironically named 'Happy Valleys' around the city fringe. It was a similar story in other major cities across the country. Many went 'on the track', joining a mass movement of itinerants, mostly men, across the rural and remote interior of the continent. Often without money and with vast tracks of open country before them, they secretly boarded moving goods or passenger trains to get to the next settlement, always hoping for an elusive job or sustenance from the local police. This was known as 'jumping the rattler'. It was both illegal and dangerous; jumpers continually faced the risk of injury or arrest. Kylie Tennant had attempted it briefly, wearing purpose-made trousers, and found negotiating moving trains extremely difficult.[15] Bee, attired in a dress and stockings, but with years of experience in negotiating moving vehicles, soon became adept at jumping trains, sometimes alone but often in the company of others. The combination of risk and movement was exhilarating. But her steady progress northwards stalled when she was arrested on a train travelling between Bundaberg and Townsville, in the small town of Rosedale. In the company of three men—Darkie, Ron and Harold—she was escorted at gunpoint to a lockup. After discussing the situation with her companions, they decided against knocking the sergeant out with a pumpkin and enjoyed a good meal and a night's rest instead. After being returned to Bundaberg for their trial, Bee spent her time writing in her cell while listening to Darkie playing the mouth organ next door. In the morning the sergeant's wife ironed her dress so she could make a good impression on the magistrate. It appears to have worked. 'Facing him am discharged but the boys get seven days which is hard. They are decent fellows. Leave them sitting sadly on the grass.' Unfortunately, the arrest was picked up by the local media and reported in the interstate papers under the heading 'Bee Miles Puts Night in Hell'.[16] Actually she had passed her evening quite pleasantly. The article also claimed she was arrested en route to Port Moresby in New Guinea. This was possibly a deliberate attempt by Bee to conceal her real destination. She was headed for the Torres Strait.

At the same time more of Bee's own pieces were appearing in Queensland newspapers. One she described as a 'bad article' was bought by the *North Queensland Register* for a guinea. She used the money to dye her dress black to prevent being spotted jumping trains. The article, which was an extract from her travel writing, describes being apprehended when she fell asleep on the roof of a moving train outside Rockhampton. She was arrested and discharged. Undeterred, she jumped a goods train and rode on top of the water tank, jumping off at each station and hiding in the grass. Eventually she was spotted by the fireman but rather than arresting her he invited her into the engine compartment, where, to her delight, he let her drive the train. Unfortunately, the experience was cut short when she fell down an ash pit during a stop. After that she rode inside the train, hidden under the seat by some passengers who also gave her some money. At the station, the ticket collector offered to let her go in exchange for sex: something, she mused, that had happened dozens of times since she had left Sydney.

By now Bee had perfected the skill of rattler jumping. She thought the drivers and guards were often aware she was on the train but deliberately chose to ignore her. Occasionally drivers would spot her and slow down to let her board. She kept moving forward, often joining groups of men, leaping off the trains before each station and climbing on again as the trains pulled out. Bee liked their company: 'Sometimes I sit on the truck with them and we laugh and chatter as the train rattles on.' For all his faults, she conceded, 'the average man can be very good company and very good fun.'[17] At Innisfail she was forced to hop off a moving train backwards as the police entered one of the carriages in the middle of the night. The police gave chase, and she was caught with one of her companions, a man called Charles. The others had escaped. They were arrested and spent the remainder of the night in the cells. In the morning she was lucky to be before 'a pleasant young magistrate. Look as if butter wouldn't melt in my mouth and am convicted and discharged. Poor Charles is given three days which is unfair because I was doing just as he was.' Abandoning Charles to his fate and giving up on the goods trains, she wrangled a lift in a car with 'a splendid chatty driver one side and a beautiful Greek lad on the other'. After stopping briefly for a drink at the Fisher Falls Hotel, she rode in comfort on to Cairns.

———

Compared to the recent weeks of rough travel, gaol cells and police pursuits, Bee's stay in Cairns was luxurious. William had sent her some money and she used it to find a room and a bath. Though initially she was not enamoured of this slow-paced, tropical town with its wide streets and the smell of ripened mangoes in the air, she liked its people. In a mood of uncharacteristic tolerance, she struck up friendships with her fellow lodgers at the boarding house and even lunched with a tea-leaf reader who told her she would have a love affair. She developed a crush on the captain of the Salvation Army band and tried to lure him into conversation during Sunday night concerts on Abbott Street. She liked the local picture theatre, the Tropical, and the architecture of the wooden homes, which reminded her of the South Sea novels of Somerset Maugham and Joseph Conrad. But most impressive of all was the fact that Cairns had a 'Malay Town', something she had never experienced before. Apart from lunching with locals and trying to find a passage further north, she spent her free time at the local newspaper *The Cairns Post*. She haunted its premises for two weeks, 'getting in everyone's way', solving crossword puzzles and 'helping' the staff with proofreading. On her last night she slept on the top of the huge paper rolls, while the 'press roars publication, publication, publication'. The rest of the evening was spent annoying the printers in the stereotype room. In the morning, with the two obliging and no doubt relieved printers carrying her bags, she went down to the harbour to try to persuade the captain of a departing boat, the *Wandana*, to take her to Thursday Island. Her money was almost gone; she only had enough to reach Cooktown. She sat on the dock. It was seven o'clock in the morning and the world was quiet: 'the hills are blue and the birds flap quietly by'. Her mood was subdued. She was tired, 'such a long way I've come', and she was lonely. She tried to raise her spirits by repeating excerpts from C.S. Forester's novel *Brown on Resolution* but was interrupted by a group of unemployed men who came to use the tap on the wharf to wash. They invited her to breakfast where they dined on fresh bread and bacon fat. After she returned to her post on the wharf to 'heave my beatitudes at the water':

> Blessed am I for I have few friends
> Blessed am I for I am broke
> Blessed am I for I am healthy.[18]

When the *Wandana* eventually arrived, Bee quickly leapt on board while it was busy docking. After filching some pineapple from the galley and annoying the stewards, she was offered a stretcher on the deck but insisted on a mattress instead. When they arrived at Cooktown, she remained on board and hid in the lifeboat intending to stowaway until Thursday Island. She had never attempted it before, but after enduring several hours in such a cramped space she abandoned it and moved into a cabin to write. Eventually she was spotted and evicted by the crew onto the wharf. Cooktown was depressing. 'The place is dead, streets in poor condition and verandas falling down, weeds on the wharf and desolation everywhere.' Worse still, there was no newspaper to buy her articles. She visited the former editor of the now-defunct *Cooktown Independent*, who told her that with a population of 500 a paper was not viable. The town's only redeeming feature was a 'Mrs Kenny', who had a beautiful and powerful contralto voice. Bee spent the day at the house of a local priest, who paid her ten shillings to help his housekeeper, after which she promptly fell ill with a fever for three days. When everything seemed at its worst, suddenly her luck changed. She met a tin miner named Neil Jenkins.

Jenkins came from a well-known tin mining family and had a camp at Mount Romeo. He nursed Bee back to health and bought her ticket to Thursday Island on the next boat. She described him as a 'bosker man', and when he invited her to visit his mine, she jumped at the chance. She was given a horse and they set out on a 50-kilometre journey accompanied by an Indigenous man, introduced as Yorkie, who worked for Jenkins. They were soon joined by a second man, George Watkin, who was leading packhorse laden with goods for outlying homes. In train with George were eight local Indigenous people—men, women and children. Initially, Bee enjoyed the ride, making friends with Kathleen, a young girl she described as a 'half-caste', riding with her ahead of the group, pretending they were scouts. But she wasn't a natural in the saddle and the blisters she developed were starting to hurt. They rode all day and into the night, moving through creeks and over boulders, the horses using their sense of smell to stay on the track, with no light but the fireflies. Eventually they arrived and Bee fell into bed exhausted. The next day she explored the settlement she described as three 'humpies' and an Aboriginal camp. The humpies consisted of a bedroom, sitting room and kitchen with an open fireplace that ran the width of the room. One was a neat and tidy structure occupied by a Cornish couple, the Roskillys.[19] She enjoyed a glorious naked swim in the local creek and a demonstration of dynamiting by Neil, whose vernacular language she greatly admired. The ants, whose bites were vicious, were like 'bloomin' hansom cabs', while his favourite oath was 'damn him from arse-hole to breakfast time'. Bee thought it was 'virile'. She spent her days being fussed over by the Roskillys and cared for by Neil but grew restless. After borrowing a horse, she set off for the long trek back to Cooktown, with Neil wisely deciding at the last minute to accompany her. Her horse-riding skills had not improved and during the journey she fell off her mount; she was knocked unconscious and also badly bruised down one side. After spending two days in Cooktown, Bee and Neil returned to Mount Romeo.

After spending a few days watching the tin being extracted and packed for shipment, Bee prepared to return to Cooktown to meet the *Wandana*, which would be arriving en route to Thursday Island. There were no vegetables at Mount Romeo and her skin had broken out in a rash. Before they left, Neil took her for a final excursion into the surrounding bush. During the ride she was nearly choked when a vine wrapped around her neck, tightening even further when her horse reared up. She had to be cut loose. Back in Cooktown she spent her time reading Ion Idriess novels[20] and playing dice in the bar of the West Coast Hotel. Neil had given her a substantial sum of money—enough to 'last for several hundred miles'. Bee gave few details about the exact nature of their relationship. She admitted that she had been 'loved a little' by him but claimed that the tea-leaf reader's prediction back in Cairns had not come true. It was time to move on and they parted on good terms. Accompanied by her generous benefactor and a group of wellwishers from the West Coast, she finally boarded the *Wandana* for Thursday Island. Five years after Bee's visit, Neil Jenkins would also become the focus of national media attention. In 1939 he made headlines when the body of a local miner was found dead after lying in the bush for a week. Around his toe was a torniquet and beside him a newspaper, with a note scribbled in charcoal over the page: 'Bitten by big brown snake. About done for. I leave everything to Neily Jenkins'. Neil's own death was equally horrendous. He died in 1953 in a truck accident after being pinned beside the dead driver all night. He was seventy years old.

———

Bee knew very little about the Torres Strait before she arrived. She had imagined a tropical paradise, free from the strictures of civilisation, where she could wander along the beach, wearing a sarong and performing the 'stomach dance' for the 'TI push'. The reality was very different. While the island's cultural and ethnic make-up was richly diverse, social divisions were rigid, with the white minority firmly in control of the rest of the population.

Racial restrictions permeated every social interaction. Torres Strait Islanders were subject to control under the *Aboriginal's Protection and Restriction of the Sale of Opium Act* and were not permitted to live on Thursday Island. Pacific Islanders were controlled by the *Pacific Islanders Act* and visiting crew members had to sleep on board ship. The rest of the islands were native reserves and entry was prohibited except for official visitors.[21] White residents were ostracised and denied employment if they associated with local Asian or mixed-race families. Bee was quick to fall out of favour: 'The white set will almost go to the length of waging a jehad of sorts against any breaker of its social laws. It refuses to speak to me.'[22] It was a very different picture than the one painted by Ernestine Hill, who also visited Thursday Island in the early 1930s. She described it as a colourful, happy and harmonious community: 'thanks to the persistent activities of Christian missioners, pearlers and protectors of aborigines, the islands have been civilised and colonised, a crown of wealth to Queensland . . . a Venice of the tropics.'[23]

After a few uncomfortable days Bee splurged her last £4 on a passage to Darwin with a boat called the *Marella*, which was heading to Singapore. When she inspected it, she was delighted to find a grand piano in the saloon and planned to make a little money during the trip by performing a concert. She was playing better than she had for a long time, having practised in hotels at every opportunity as she made her way north. But it would be a month until the *Marella* would depart, so in the meantime she found lodgings with a Chinese family. In this small and tightly controlled settlement, Bee quickly came under the scrutiny of the local authorities. When she went to consult a local doctor, he lectured her on the dangers of white women being raped by 'dark men'. She described him as a self-appointed 'protector of women's purity' and a member of the Society for the Diffusion of Useful Knowledge—the SDUK.[24] Arguing that the reverse was true and that white men were more likely to be predators, she was also outraged by his interference in her private life. 'I went to consult him on a health matter and he poked his finger into a pie I made myself . . . I make lovely pies and there's only one man who may finger it [sic].'

The encounter had angered her and triggered memories that were always sitting just below the surface, resulting in a vehement attack on the duplicity of doctors:

> The medical profession is the least gentlemanly of any bar the legal. Even the police warn prisoners that anything they say may be used as evidence against them; but consider the doctor who is examining the person suspected of insanity. The medico does not warn him that his words may put him into that hell on earth, a Mental Hospital, but under the usually false pretences of being able to help him, will worm his way into the patient's mind, unearth his secrets and declare him insane. What gentleman will poke his nose into a man's or a woman's private affairs? . . . For example two doctors who indulge in the pleasant pastime of reading private letters when the proper recipient is not in a position to retaliate . . . Unfortunately for the truth doctors have the capacity to assume a thick veneer of breeding and one must incise deeply before the truth is discovered.[25]

The fear of being returned to a psychiatric facility, 'that hell on earth', which never left her, was now bubbling to the surface. She would have been acutely aware that on Thursday Island, as a single white woman, with no legitimate purpose, her presence would also have caused anxiety and suspicion amongst the locals.

Eventually she found some distraction and more agreeable company at a 'coloured dance' she attended. Everyone was polite and 'no one put the hard word' on her. She danced with a shy and handsome pupil teacher of Torres Strait and Malaysian heritage, played games, and watched the Japanese divers who had dressed for the occasion in blue-and-white patterned kimonos. For these transgressions, she was promptly evicted from her lodgings the following day. She found new accommodation with Mrs Chin Soon, who had six daughters. She liked them immediately and admired their mother's relaxed attitude towards child-rearing. It was so different, she thought, from the way white mothers repressed and coddled their children, preventing them from gaining independence until they were much older. She was sure that this increased the rate of mental illness. She played for them every day on Mrs Chin Soon's excellent Victor piano.

At last, the long month was over and the *Marella* was preparing to depart. Bee's reputation was increasingly disreputable, with the island's white population 'becoming a bit narked about my low habits'. In a final act of rebellion she attended another 'coloured dance' the night before she left. She was soon approached by 'a man of religion', who tried to get her to leave by calling the police. She refused and told him she too 'had dark blood and therefore have a perfect right to be here'. The police sergeant arrived but she ignored him and was left in peace to dance all night with the handsome pupil teacher. Her friends gave her a farewell dinner and she was taken by launch out to Black Rock where the *Marella* was anchored waiting to depart.

———

The two-day trip to Darwin was dull. Bee was unable to perform a concert because the piano she had inspected previously was in the first-class section. In second class she played a less grand instrument before a crowd of talkers and was hesitant to ask for payment. She passed her time raiding the pantry of the first-class kitchen and playing games with a young man she met on the deck. Arriving in Darwin, Bee immediately made for the train. She had spent her money on the boat ticket and so was back to rattler jumping. Now she was in a carriage, hopping up and down on one leg, trying to work out what to do. Eventually she scampered onto one of the trucks but was spotted and thrown off. Having no alternative, she headed for the road that would take her towards Alice Springs, nearly 1500 kilometres away. Bee sat on a lonely stretch of highway waiting for a car. She tried playing patience to pass the time, but the cards blew away, so she wrote in her journal instead. A young woman on a bicycle stopped for a chat. She was named Melba, because the famous singer was playing on the gramophone when she was born. Sometime after Melba left a truck pulled up with the bad news that no cars would be leaving Darwin for several days. The driver took her to Melba's place where she was made welcome and given a bed.[26] Bee was quick to notice the racial divisions and, out of deference to Melba's family, the Dargies, who had let her stay without 'a hint for me to leave', didn't seek out the company of the Indigenous people employed at the family homestead. She had run out of money and was dependent on other people's generosity. After failing to sell her articles to the local paper, *The Northern Standard,* she went to the police to ask for a ticket to Katherine, but they refused because she wasn't a resident. The next few days were spent in a fruitless search for a seat on a plane. Eventually a lift in a car was secured for three days' time. Sensing that she couldn't stay at the Dargies' any longer, she slept on the table of the local hotel. It's not clear why she left the Dargies but there are hints in the manuscript that she may have transgressed racial boundaries. Antipathy or prejudice towards Indigenous people, she noted afterwards, was the very definition of irrationality.

The hotel where Bee was staying, the Victoria, was run by Mrs Christina Gordon, known as Ma, who was famous throughout the Territory. Bee was delighted to learn that she had travelled across Australia on donkey, camel and horse. She was, Bee thought, a true woman of the world, who only laughed when she heard that a man had barged into Bee's room the night before and was still there snoring hard in the next bed. There seemed to be a mutual fondness and Bee was allowed to stay free of charge. Finally, she was on the road once more, heading for the tiny settlement of Grove Hill and the Gaden homestead. The Gadens were noted buffalo shooters, with a butchery on the property. Bee admired the independence of the children, who taught her some bush skills. Ernestine Hill also visited the Gadens and made similar observations.[27] Beginning to doubt she would ever make it home, and perhaps inspired by the butchering activity around her, Bee outlined provisions for the dismemberment and distribution of her body parts: her skull to be erected on the radiator of Police Commissioner MacKay's car and her heart canned and placed in the Casualty Ward of Sydney Hospital.[28] After spending the night with the Gadens where she slept on buffalo hide, she joined the train and rode with the engine driver to Birdum, where her ticket expired. At the Birdum Hotel she enticed the local mailman into giving her a lift to Daly Waters, where she was given accommodation by the Pearce family, who, she claimed, were hanging onto their property like grim death. From there, in the company of several of the Pearce children and an Indigenous man named Prentiss, she travelled by truck to Newcastle Waters, where a silent Scottish policeman directed her to the home-stead of Lance Lewis.

Newcastle Waters was, and remains, a huge pastoral property ranging over 10,000 square kilometres. John Lewis, Lance's father, had acquired the lease in 1895. He was both a pastoralist and a politician and served in the South Australian Legislative Council. He was a member of the Australian Geographical Society and the Aborigines' Friends Association along with Ngarrindjeri author and inventor David Unaipon.[29] This may have explained the less rigid racial conditions Bee observed during her stay of six days. There were several other guests, including an anthropologist who was 'studying' local Indigenous people. Bee was sceptical, claiming that it would take years to understand the complexity of their belief systems. But she was also observing: watching the graceful way the Indigenous women crossed the yard and comparing them to statues of Greek goddesses. She admired the way they went about their domestic work, their calm and efficient manner and their indiffer-ence to her presence. 'The Abos. [sic] don't take the slightest notice of me though I'm the only white woman here. Some women might be piqued at their indifference.'[30]

The apparent racial tolerance Bee witnessed at Newcastle Waters was very different from the broader reality of race relations in the Northern Territory. White people were in the minority and utterly dependent on Indigenous labour for survival. But they also controlled the economy and the law. All Indigenous people were subject to the *Northern Territory Aboriginal Ordinance Act*, which gave the chief protector control over every aspect of their lives. In 1934 the protector was Dr Cecil Cook, who was also the chief medical officer—Bee would have seen this as the worst possible conflation of medical and legal authority. While Cook had introduced some innovative public health measures and had studied anthropology under Professor Radcliffe Brown (a frequent visitor to Pakie's Club), he was also subject to the same overriding anxiety about the vulnerability of white Australians and the proximity of Asia that was shared by the broader population.[31] Ernestine Hill's depictions of fragile white societies struggling against a surging racial tide in the Territory in the 1930s were typical of this view: 'Already the white children are far in the minority at all Territory schools. Already the steady increase of coloured and half-breed populations threatens an empty country with the begetting of one of the most illogical and inbred races in the world.'[32] But Hill, it should be noted, was subtly critical of Cook and his practices. Under the motto 'breed out the colour', Cook oversaw the systematic, forced removal of mixed-descent children from their families by placing them in government institutions. Indigenous women of mixed descent could not marry without Cook's consent, giving him an almost god-like control over the racial make-up of future generations. Indigenous people who were deemed free of mixed ancestry, known as 'full bloods' were isolated into reserves, where access and contact were strictly controlled. Cook's policies on mixed-race populations were described as biological absorption. The reality was a comprehensive eugenics program that was replicated in Western Australia, as well as other parts of the country.[33] Bee believed that the antipathy of whites towards the Indigenous people she had witnessed was based on fear and a false sense of superiority. The more she travelled through the Territory, the more convinced she was that this fear was entrenched, and that most people were incapable of 'arguing themselves free of it'. She would return to this theme repeatedly in her future writing.

After six days of the Lewises' hospitality, herding goats and playing with the children, the heavily laden mail truck arrived and, with Bee sitting on the back, it set out for Alice Springs, stopping at more stations along the way. The country was greener due to recent rains, and she saw water in the creeks for the first time since she'd left Darwin. During a brief stop at a goldmine she met two cameleers, an 'Afghan' and a 'Baluch', who offered her a place by their fire. She admired their turbans, underneath which was a 'shimmering, gold-cloth, fez-like cap'. They produced an even more impressive specimen, a dazzling combination of gold, red and blue. Back on the road once more they travelled on slowly until they arrived at the Barrow Creek Hotel. After a quiet word from the mailman George, Bee was given free board and lodging in exchange for doing the washing up. Sitting on her bed at five o'clock the next morning, she examined her clothing: a green tartan shirt given to her by a man in Tennant Creek, over which she wore her thin cotton dress, a light sweater, and her beloved cestus. It was, she said, as cold as charity.

But the charity she had received on this stretch of her trip had been anything but cold. She had been fed and housed at each stage of her long journey across the Northern Territory. Somewhat surprisingly, her presence as a single, white, itinerant female did not create the same levels of anxiety as it had in the Torres Strait. In turn, her own anxiety was considerably lessened by the dearth of police. If people found her presence strange or her behaviour odd, they didn't seem to show it. In fact, there was a kind of acceptance that was reminiscent of bohemian culture. George, the indefatigable mailtruck driver, had put up with her singing the entire journey. Her repertoire consisted of around 150 songs, including jazz, grand opera, Gilbert and Sullivan, and the sacred songs her father had taught her from his days in the St Mary's Cathedral choir. By the time they were approaching Alice Springs, she had subjected her fellow travellers to all of them. Every now and then George would distract Bee by giving her chewing gum or cigarettes. When she told him that she had inherited her grandmother's love of singing, he replied that it was a pity she hadn't inherited her fine contralto voice as well.

In Alice Springs Bee was hosted by two local women, and she played her best piano for them in return for their hospitality. The next morning she was given ten shillings and a ticket by a young man and hoisted onto the train 'with clothing and brushes flying everywhere'. Her ticket took her as far as Oodnadatta, where she would face more rattler jumping, her finances now depleted. At Oodnadatta, in the traditional lands of the Arabana, the local policeman directed her to the United Aboriginal Mission, where the missionary gave her a bed and a breakfast of two eggs and tea. It was the first meal she'd had since leaving Alice Springs. The missionary also informed her that a car was going south and so, with her companions Jim and Wally, she set out for Maree across the rocky gibber country. At Maree she tried unsuccessfully to hide in a coal truck but was driven inside by the cold, discovered, and thrown off the train at Hawker. Eventually, after being ejected from another train halfway to Peterborough, she spent the night in a police cell. In the morning she met a fruiterer who offered her a lift to Adelaide where she surrendered herself to the Women's Police. They gave her a meal but insulted her in the process by calling her a liar when she insisted she had been at university. Rather than risking any further antagonism, she spent the night sleeping in a parked car and left the city in the early hours of the morning.

She was getting closer to Sydney now, but there was still a long way to go, and she was worried about having to pass through Melbourne, given her experience twelve months before. The police had promised that she would be arrested on sight if she returned.

She was also having trouble getting a lift. Each car that stopped told her to wait for the next one. The weather was 'piercingly cold'. Finally, a driver stopped but the reprieve was short-lived. His windscreen shattered and they were forced to drive with the icy rain in their faces, discarding shards of broken glass on the way. Reaching Kingston, and having no alternative, she went to the local police station where she was given a meal and a bed. And so it continued with one lift worse than the other until she reached the coastal town of Port Fairy in Victoria. After approaching the local hotel for a free bed, Bee was reported to the police. She gave them a false name and justified her presence by reading them excerpts from her manuscript, careful to leave out any references to Melbourne. They seemed satisfied by the demonstration and gave her a bed in the cells and some extra blankets.

In a rare turn of events, two women picked her up on the way to Camperdown. It didn't go well. After asking them politely if she could smoke, they told her it was a dirty filthy habit. 'If I saw my daughter smoking,' the older woman said, 'I'd smack her in the mouth.' After Bee responded weakly that her mother had smoked, the lectures continued. She soon left them and immediately caught a lift with a driver who entertained her with his extensive knowledge of local history. But he did make her get out at Colac and walk the length of the town, worried that the shopkeepers might spot him with a young woman in his car if they drove through together. At last she arrived in Melbourne and went straight to her hide-out at Osborne House in Fitzroy, where the obliging Mrs Meagher gave her a bed.

———

Bee stayed in Melbourne for twelve hours, enough for a sleep and a quick catch-up with some friends in the maids' department of Myer's. She quickly picked up a lift to Albury, hoping to cross the border as soon as possible. After crossing over the Murray River into New South Wales and leaving her fear of the Victorian police behind, Bee sat and waited for another lift. As she did, she mused about the definition of right and wrong and her thoughts turned yet again to 'P', who had argued that nothing was clear-cut. Suicide was legal in Japan but considered a criminal act in Australia. Wearing a bathing suit in the street was illegal in Cronulla but permitted in Collaroy. Murder was wrong but war was sanctioned. No one could really define the difference between right and wrong, she concluded, particularly 'Mental Specialists'. Her musings were cut short when a young family picked her up. They took her home and gave her a bath, a meal and a bed, and soon she was on the track to Sydney. After a succession of lifts, including one with a one-armed driver who drove on the wrong side of the road at an alarming speed, Bee was on the last stretch. Now the drivers who picked her up were starting to recognise her. 'You're a long way from your territory,' one told her as he pulled up beside her outside Yass. Normally such recognition would fill her with apprehension, but now she was almost overcome with joy—she was getting close to home.

Bee had been away for six months; her clothes were in tatters, her dress covered in cigarette burns and her shoes worn through. She had traversed huge tracts of country, learned to jump the rattler, visited the tropics and conquered the desert. But now she was tired and homesick. She vowed to herself that when she finally made it back to Sydney, she would stay home 'and be respectable'. The reason for the trip had been to avoid a return to Kenmore. Now she needed to work out a way to be able to remain in Sydney while staying out of trouble. She vowed to change: 'Shall never shout "hello" to newsboys and policeman; shall never jump on a moving tram; and shall never poke my nose into Sydney Hospital however alluring the ether and iodoform breeze.'[34] Riding triumphantly down Parramatta Road, past the university and Central Station she treated her companion to one last song—this time one of her own, based on Kipling's 'Prodigal Son':

Here come I to my own again,
Chased and worried and jailed again,
I think I'll start to be good again,
And give up my old, wild ways.

Now she was back in Sydney she would collect her travel notes and develop them into 'I Leave in a Hurry', her second manuscript: 'dedicated to P because he filled my thoughts while I was away'. The manuscript, written in neat cursive script, is full of notations and explanatory footnotes of people, places and language. The narrative, with its lively picaresque style and literary and classical allusions is reminiscent of Furphy's *Such is Life*, but the narrative voice is closer to Langley's Steve in the *Pea-Pickers*. Like Steve, the character Bee presents is self-deprecating, never quite mastering the world in which she is travelling. She is constantly falling off horses or down ash pits, getting spotted by police and locked up in the cells. She takes an obvious delight in vernacular language and lampooning pomposity and social pretensions. Although the manuscript suffers from a lack of scrupulous editing, particularly in the long diatribes on communism or the hypocrisy of conventional society, its publication would have made an interesting contribution to the travel literature of the time.

The version that was eventually submitted to the publisher Frank Johnson was significantly different. It was written in third person, initially titled 'She Leaves in a Hurry', but then changed to 'For We Are Young and Free'. It is incomplete, only covering the trip as far as Brisbane. It may have been provided as a sample chapter. The introduction had been expanded and included additional information on the reasons for the protagonist's sudden departure from Sydney. She was facing gaol on charges of taxi fare evasion. On two separate occasions, taxi drivers had demanded sex and she had abandoned the cabs. She knew she would not be believed, so she would leave town instead. It was Bee's way of addressing the inequities of the justice system. Life, she claimed, in her introduction, was not worth living but what little joy that could be derived from it was worth celebrating. She had also decided that she would have to fly alone:

> Bee knows no one who would go on a walkabout with her. She has gone her way alone for some years now and loneliness is understood and appreciated. At first it scared her and she wandered far and wide looking for someone who could see her point of view. Several people said they did but, on being put to the test, were found to be wanting in any sort of wits. She came to the conclusion that most people have no comprehension of behaviour, desires, experience, ideas, and standards other than their own; very little of their own and of themselves generally. So that was that and she is content . . . Loneliness is good: for some at any rate. It gives one time to make decisions and reach conclusions, time to know oneself. Anyway she prefers going alone. Bar the delight she takes in pleasing one other person only in this world, she takes delight in pleasing herself. When she is not with him she goes her own way. Whose way should she go? The way of a lady? Bee was born one but she falls far short of the average man's conception of one.[35]

This version of the manuscript, which also remained unpublished, was 'dedicated to herself because she went by herself'. At some stage, it is unclear when, she had discovered that 'P', the man she had fallen so heavily in love with, had a wife and four sons.[36] Though it is likely that the relationship was already over by then, she had remained in love with him until she found out that, unlike her, he was the marrying kind after all.

9

Grand Schemes

'I can't always do as I please. I would very much like to climb
to the top of Queen Victoria's statue in Queen's Square and
put a pipe in her mouth but my fear of the police stops me.'

Bee Miles, 'I Go on a Wild Goose Chase', p. 54

Buried within the Kenmore Hospital case notes is a brief letter
from the inspector general of mental hospitals, Charles Hogg, to
Superintendent Moffitt. He wanted to know on what basis Bee had
been recommended for release from hospital supervision. Moffitt
responded that she had presented, as requested on 25 April 1935,
and had asked to be discharged.[1] He saw no basis for retaining her
further. Either there had been an improvement in her behaviour or
Moffitt was at last resigned to the fact that Bee was 'unalterable'.
Things were about to change for Bee, though perhaps not in the way
her psychiatrists had hoped.

In late 1935 Bee made a dramatic announcement. She decided
she would go to London and Paris. Bernard Hesling recalled 'all
intellectual Sydney was agog not with speculation as to how the
London bobby would cope with her traffic hopping, but rather
what would come out of her summit with [George Bernard] Shaw

and [H.G.] Wells—for we had no doubt that they would take her into their aging hearts'.[2] The only drawback to this grand plan was her financial situation—she was broke again. Lying in bed at night and considering her options, she came up with a 'glorious' plan to travel to Tennant Creek and open a school for the children of miners, who had been drawn to the remote settlement by the recent discovery of gold. It was as improbable as it was impractical. She had no teaching qualifications, having been dismissed from kindergarten teacher training after only a few months of study. Perhaps she was thinking of her own early education at private day schools and conveniently forgetting her earlier claim that she hated children. Even if she brushed all that aside, she didn't have the capital required for such a project.

Undeterred by reality, on a cold October morning in 1935, Bee walked determinedly up Macleay Street in Kings Cross to commence the 3,200-kilometre journey to Tennant Creek. It was 4 a.m. and the lights glistened on the plane trees lining the empty street. All was quiet apart from a lone taxi looking for fares. She was tempted to hail it, but she had no money. A milk lorry pulled up beside her. She was surprised as they didn't usually stop for her. 'Where are you going?' the driver asked her sarcastically. 'Bourke?' To his amazement she answered, 'Yes!' and climbed on board before he could change his mind. Sometime later she was standing on the corner of Regent and George Streets in the city, examining her belongings—a rug, a bag and a small port (suitcase). With all this luggage, there would be no jumping on bumper bars; she would have to be a lady on this trip. She 'hated being a lady'.[3]

Initially, Bee was lucky with rides, reaching Lawson in the Blue Mountains quite quickly, where she was given some tea and bread and butter by the local nuns. Afterwards she sat in the gutter, filled with remorse, and repeated a passage from the Norman Douglas novel *South Wind* on the evils of charity.

Douglas described charity as a destructive and artificial practice that upset the national equilibrium 'by keeping alive an incredible number of people who ought to be dead', leading to a deterioration of humanity as a whole. It was an argument that had considerable currency throughout the late nineteenth and early twentieth centuries, riding in tandem with other eugenic ideas, including, somewhat ironically for Bee, the management of the mentally 'unfit'.[4] After repeating the tract solemnly to herself three times, Bee decided it would have no effect on her determination to 'forage' en route and promptly accepted another ride to Orange, pushing further west towards her destination. She filled in time between rides writing in her notebooks, describing towns she passed through and musing on one of her favourite themes—the foibles and virtues of 'the average man'. This figure would feature continually in Bee's writing, in the manifestos she developed and in the speeches she gave. Occasionally the definition of the average man would expand to include women, but for the most part he was male. He usually represented the worst aspects of humanity, but he also possessed some redeeming features, if he was able to free himself from the strictures of polite or civilised society. He could also be 'good fun' and enjoyable company, provided he hadn't joined the professional class—'the cads' who became doctors and lawyers and were bound by middle-class pretensions. Sometimes, Bee wrote, she 'liked him awfully'. Unfortunately, and inevitably, she lamented, the men in her company developed passionate ideas, which she found nauseating. 'Passion is for women, a man if he is to be a woman's superior, must be cold and restrained.' She knew this would mean the likelihood that she would end up alone, 'a repressed and savage spinster'. She didn't mind being a spinster but she didn't like the idea of being repressed and savage.

Bee landed in Bathurst, which she described as an anti-charity town. She'd been here before and had been sent to a religious charity by the police. She had been offered a cup of tea and three slices of toast, while the men next to her were 'wolfing down stew and grilled chops'. Afterwards she had slept in a bed infested with fleas. Her experience reflected what was occurring on a broader scale across the country. Officially economic recovery from the Great Depression began in 1932, but for many people, unemployment, homelessness and displacement were still a bitter reality. On this second journey across Australia, Bee once again joined unemployed, itinerant men on the track and made consistent use of the limited welfare opportunities that were available, including the Red Cross and the Salvation Army. While charities went some way to fill the gap left by inadequate government support for the unemployed, their services were often conditional upon adherence to the institution's codes and values.[5] Frank Huelin, writing of his experiences on the track in the same period Bee was travelling, described the rituals involved in obtaining food and shelter at the Salvation Army:

> We joined the choruses of Washing the Blood and Beautiful Words. Sat unmoved through the major's vehement appeal to come to the 'penitent stool'. Listened to a female Salvationist's account of the pleasure to be found In the Arms of Jesus, said 'amen' and 'halleluiah' as the 'methos' and 'plonkos' staggered to the 'penitent stool' to earn bed and breakfast for the next few hours . . . Then came the free supper, the bait for which hungry men hypocritically sang, prayed . . . The supper consisted of a thin, brown, barely sweetened liquid alleged to be 'cocoa'. . . the food was a very solid bun, no longer saleable even at a reduced price.[6]

It's difficult to imagine Bee praying for her supper, no matter how hungry she was. Her atheism was too firmly entrenched. But she did seek work at pubs and hotels wherever she stopped, in exchange for food and accommodation. Her efforts met with mixed success. In Dubbo, on the Western Plains, she was ejected from two pubs, but at the third she was 'welcomed with open arms'. She was given a room and two 'bounteous' meals, without having to do any work. 'Such a decent proprietor,' she wrote. 'I fancy he knows what it's like to be broke and on the road.'

In the small town of Nyngan, she found a job for two days in a pub and made friends with the female proprietor, who arranged a lift for her with two commercial travellers. They gave her a lift to Bourke, where to her surprise she met the 'friendliest blokes in the police force'. Rather than the usual close questioning about her purpose for being in town, they arranged for her accommodation in a pub and enlisted the help of the local Country Women's Association (CWA). She took the opportunity to wash and mend her clothes and her rug, and slept early. This was not unusual. Years of institutionalised living had meant she was always in bed by 6 p.m. With characteristic precision, she noted that she had been going to bed at this hour for thirteen years, except for one hundred nights. Twenty-eight of these were spent behind the conductor, Maurice de Abravanel, during an opera season. He was a great maestro, according to Bee, and though his gestures were magnificent and sweeping, he only hit her once in the eye with his baton.[7]

———

From Bourke, where the temperature was 110 degrees Fahrenheit (43 degrees Celsius), the country grew increasingly arid and barren as Bee made her way in a series of trucks through to Cunnamulla in Queensland. The novelist Miles Franklin had travelled the same route up from Bourke five months earlier in April, though she travelled by train with a companion, and had been feted by the local press.[8] Bee's reception was somewhat different. In this small, remote township, where social activity was centred around local football and the races, Bee would have been an unusual sight. She was still slim and athletic but had now taken to wearing an eyeshade and dark glasses—possibly to combat a sensitivity to light, an after-effect of encephalitis lethargica. She was wearing frocks again, simple dresses she mended constantly, made from either cotton or flannelette material, because they didn't irritate her skin. She felt a little more confident on this trip, believing she had a legitimate reason to be travelling, and that made her less hesitant to approach local businesses. Up to now she had been treated well, but her luck changed when she met a man she mistook for the proprietor of a local pub and asked for a free drink of raspberry syrup. She suspected he might be drunk but took up his offer to lie down on a sofa for a sleep. Moments later the real publican appeared and promptly called the police who arrested her for vagrancy. She spent two days in a wood-walled, tin-roofed cell in stifling heat but she made good use of the time, washing and mending her clothes, playing patience and writing. Once again, her charges were dismissed by the magistrate when she faced the court, who took issue with the local police instead. Before discharging her, the magistrate had tried to dissuade her from going to Tennant Creek, telling her that the miners there 'were frightful'. Remembering the very pleasant time she had spent at Neil Jenkins' tin mine, she disagreed, so he ordered her to leave town. She was happy to comply. An unknown citizen came forward to pay her fare to Charleville. She'd already travelled over 1600 kilometres and was only halfway to her destination.

Bee's travels through the rest of western Queensland followed a similar pattern. She was often given free accommodation and meals at pubs and was treated reasonably well. When she told people her intention to travel to Tennant Creek, they didn't react with scorn or ridicule. One local merely told her 'It was a long lead'. She savoured that expression and used it frequently. The kindness she was shown made her question her own assumptions about human behaviour: 'Bias says all men are bad and that makes it hard for me to believe that they welcome me out of kindness of heart though it looks frightfully like it. Perhaps I'm due for a change of heart.'[9] Her musings were cut short when she was arrested in the tiny settlement of Blackall and put in the cells again. Initially, the arresting constable was relaxed and allowed her to play in the paddocks with his son. In the gaol she tidied all the cells and politely refused the advances of another prisoner who was locked up for drunk and disorderly. Then another, more senior, constable, equipped with large bunches of keys, appeared. His aim, she said, was 'to put the bounce into us'. It was a tactic she'd seen many times before. The charge nurses in the psychiatric hospitals would frequently jangle large bunches of keys as a sign of authority when they wanted to intimidate the patients. The constable insisted on taking her fingerprints, but she was well versed in this process too. In the foetid heat of the cells, with Bee struggling and the constable's rage rising with the temperature, she managed to produce a badly blurred and useless set of prints. In court, yet again the magistrate refused to convict, and in a final act of humiliation, the constable was ordered to pay Bee's fare to Barcaldine.

Bee was in the relative comfort of a mail car now—the only available transport—but the trip made her miserable. Although she was the only passenger, and the country 'frightfully dry and tough', the driver refused to pick up a couple of men who asked for a lift. 'I run for hire,' he told her bluntly. Her equivocation about the possibility that people might just be motivated by kindness abruptly vanished. 'Most people are miserable most of the time and when they see someone more miserable than themselves or in a quandary or wanting something they possess and can and do withhold, they feel less miserable by comparison.'[10] Eventually she arrived in Longreach and went to the police for advice. They were already aware of her presence but, rather than arresting her, they arranged accommodation at the local hospital, where she was 'looked after like a Queen Bee instead of killed like a drone'. The matron gave her a piece of mosquito netting and an old hat. Although she was tempted to stay and enjoy the comfort, she moved on, eventually arriving at Winton where she met the 'sweetest woman I know'. This unnamed woman was the proprietor of the North Gregory Hotel, famous as the site where 'Waltzing Matilda' was first played in public. Bee was so impressed with the owner that she not only tolerated her kind lecturing about her 'errant ways', she was almost persuaded to 'give them up and settle down like a lady'.

Almost, but not quite.

Bee was soon back in the 110-degree heat (43 degrees Celsius), waiting on the outskirts of town for a lift. After five hours a car appeared. 'In it are two men, but plenty of room for a sylph like me. Do they give me a lift? Though I have neither food nor water and am going the same way as they [sic], they refuse utterly. They are womanly enough to object "what would our wives say?" Blasted sissies!'[11] She had more success with 'two cheerful young squatters' in a lorry, who paid for her room and meals at Dick's Creek Hotel, where she planned to pick up the mail lorry. The driver, when he finally arrived, was reluctant to let her in the vehicle. After a brief stand-off he capitulated and she rode with him to Kynuna, where she picked up another mail lorry. This time the driver allowed her to stay in the cab while he drove through the night. The trip continued in much the same way, travelling on bumpy, empty, unsealed roads, passing scattered settlements and railway sidings in an assortment of vehicles, until she reached Cloncurry, where she was arrested for rattler jumping. After spending a fitful night in yet another stifling gaol, she awoke to find two doctors in her cell. The police sergeant had thought she might be insane because she'd been jumping the train. Not realising the irony of his question, one of the doctors asked her in hushed tones if she felt any shame at being in a police cell. She provided what she believed was an extremely rational defence:

> I try to point out that I'm full of joy at this near approach to
> equity. If I jump rattlers and the government punishes me
> for it, then the government and I are even and can start off
> again in a friendly way. That the government will develop
> beastly suspicions of me cannot be helped. That won't make
> me any worse. So that my being in a cell should occasion me
> no shame at all.[12]

The doctors were unpersuaded and, informing her that she was in a very grave position, sent her to the Cloncurry Hospital. If it was meant to be a preventative measure or a punishment, her

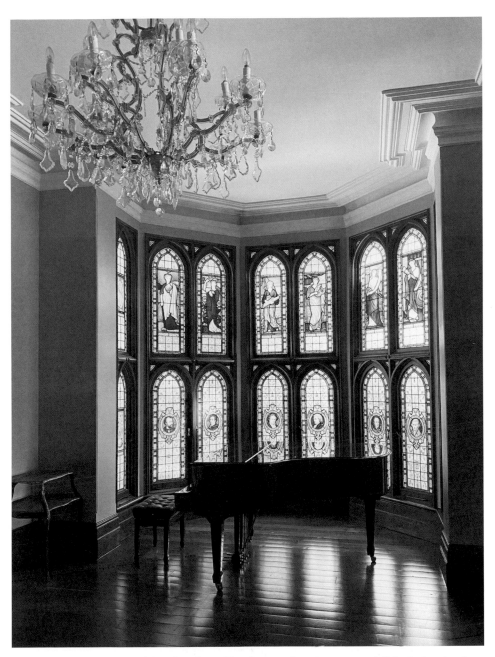

The music room at Ambleside where Bee learnt the piano as a child, sitting in the light of the many stained-glass windows. *Courtesy of Jean Rhodes*

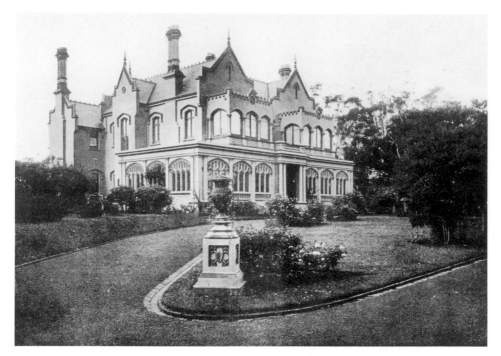

Ambleside—also known as Ashfield Castle—the home of Bee's grandparents.
Courtesy of Bill Barlow

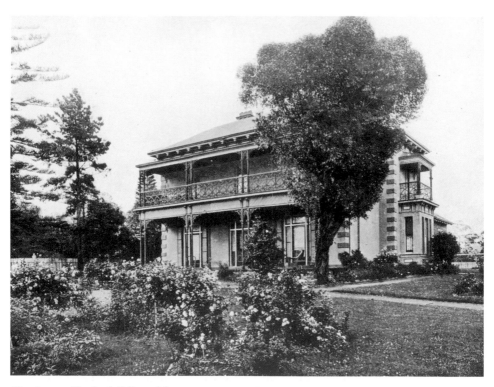

Coniston, Bee's childhood home. *Courtesy of Bill Barlow*

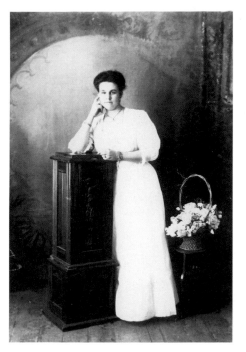

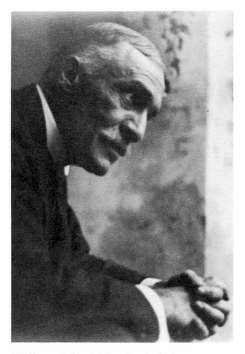

Maria Louisa Miles, Bee's mother.
Courtesy of Cathy Drew

William John Miles, Bee's father.
Courtesy of the State Library of New South Wales

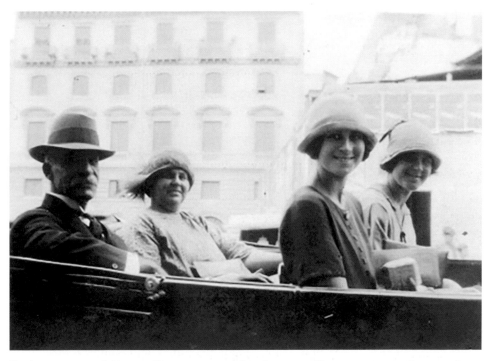

Bee's parents and sisters, Constance and Louise, on a European tour. *Courtesy of Bill Barlow*

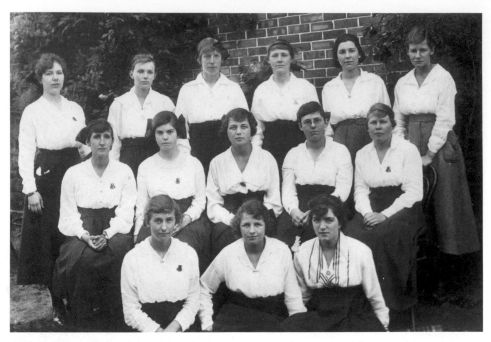

Abbotsleigh examination class, 1919. Bee is standing second from right in the back row. *Courtesy of Abbotsleigh Archives*

STRANGE MENTAL CHANGES.

Strange consequences of encephalitis lethargica (sleepy sickness) are recorded by Dr. G. A. Auden, school medical officer, Birmingham, in "The Lancet." He writes:—

"In a large number of cases which recover, the after history shows a definite change. The quiet housewife develops the temper of a shrew, or the model husband begins to neglect his home. Such effects may assume a sociological importance, for cases will probably occur in which the question of criminal responsibility is raised and an attack of encephalitis may be urged in defence of some anti-social act."

Dr. Auden gives a number of illustrative cases. A girl who was normal till she was eight, when she had an attack of sleepy sickness, became uncontrollable at the age of ten. Her mother said:— "She will go into shops and take anything. She is very destructive, and cuts up the sheets and curtains to make dolls' clothing; she also cuts up her own clothes. She set baby's hair alight with a candle, and takes her father's food from under his eyes."

"We are having many cases of encephalitis lethargica," writes a medical correspondent. "In London last week six cases were notified. About one-fourth of the people who were attacked in Birmingham in 1919-20 have shown changes in moral character. Apparently this disease will produce a good many criminals."

With sleeping accommodation for 200 passengers, and able to carry 100 tons of freight for a non-stop run of 4000 miles, an airship 900ft long has been designed by a German engineer.

Diamonds feel much colder to the tongue than paste or glass.

SLEEPY DISEASE CLAIMS ANOTHER VICTIM

In two years three lives have been lost at Forbes from encephalitis lethargica, better known as "sleeping sickness."

Latest victim was 2½-year-old Leonie Field, daughter of Mr. and Mrs. P. W. Field, of Daroobalgie (near Forbes), who died in the Forbes District Hospital on Monday.

The child had been admitted to hospital last Wednesday.

The disease often accompanies a type of influenza, a doctor states.

It results from involvement of the central nervous system, one of the early symptoms being increasing drowsiness Headache, double vision and diarrhoea are frequent accompaniments to the principle symptom of drowsiness.

During the second stage of the disease, feverishness, general weakness and stupor, with speech difficulties and twitching of the face and limbs, become evident.

The disease has the possibility of reaching epidemic proportions, it is stated.

There were two deaths from it last year at Forbes.

Now largely forgotten, from the 1920s reports about encephalitis lethargica cases appeared in the media for thirty years. The article on the left appeared in the *Newcastle Morning Herald and Miners' Advocate* in 1922, and the article on the right appeared in the *Dubbo Liberal and Macquarie Advocate* in 1951. *Trove*

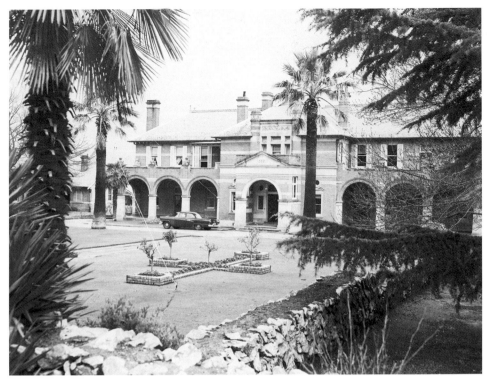

Kenmore Hospital. *Courtesy of New South Wales State Archives*

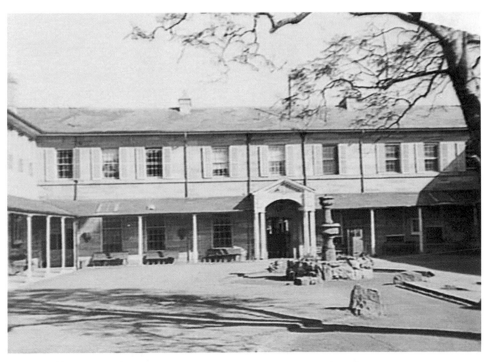

Gladesville Hospital. *Courtesy of the State Library of New South Wales*

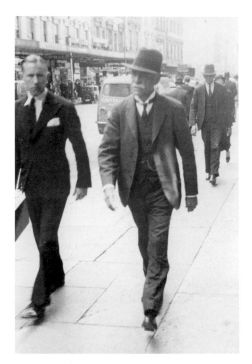

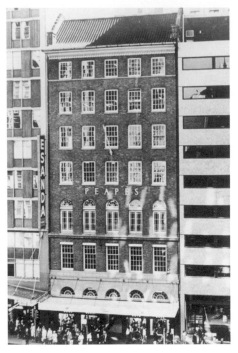

William Miles in Sydney, circa 1935—always a man on a mission.
Courtesy of Bill Barlow

Peapes department store 'For men and their sons'—its high-quality merchandise and prime location drew shoppers from across the country.
Courtesy of Matthew Miles

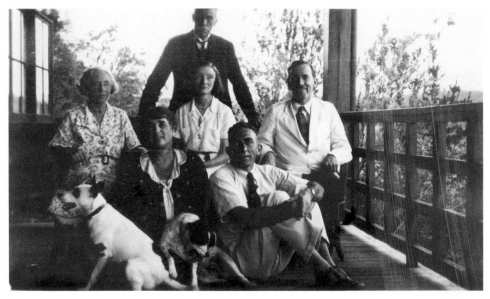

In happier times. Standing: William Miles; seated: unidentified female, Winnifred Stephensen, Inky Stephensen; seated on floor: unidentified female, Xavier Herbert.
Courtesy of the State Library of New South Wales

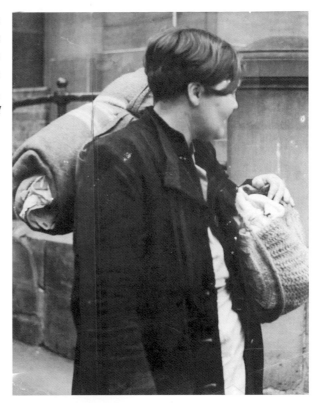

Bee sporting her swag in the city and 'upsetting the constipated snobs who travel down to town from the stuffy suburbs'. *Courtesy of News Ltd*

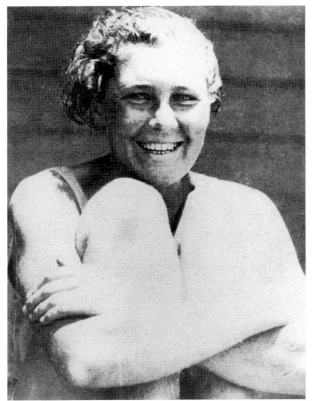

Bee Miles aged 29, young and free and swimming up and down the 'sea coast of Bohemia'. *Courtesy of Bill Barlow*

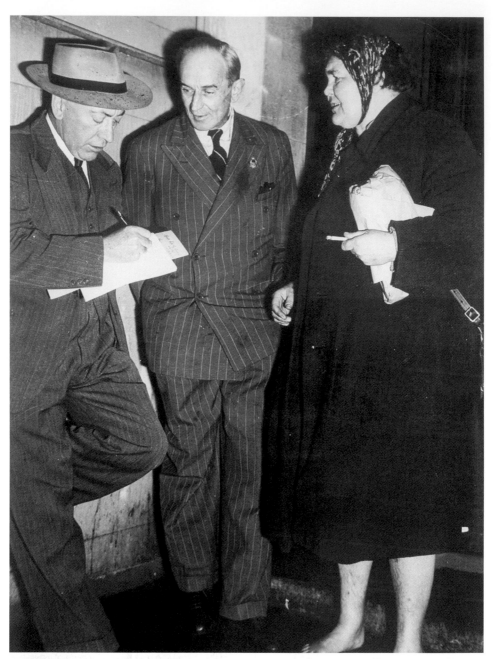

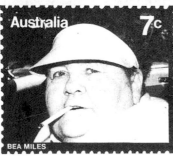

Above: Bee with Theo Walters being interviewed by a reporter. They were charged after Theo kissed Bee on the cheek while she was in the police station being charged for another offence.
Courtesy of the State Library of New South Wales

Left: *The Bulletin*'s nomination for a postage stamp proposed for the 1975 International Year for Women. *The Bulletin, 12 January, 1974*

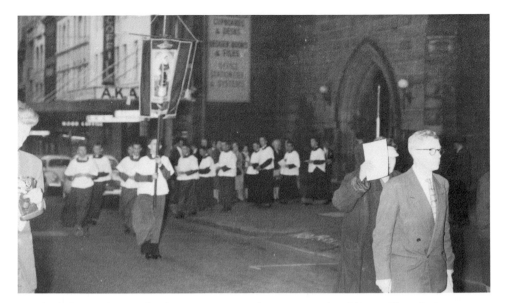

Bee hiding in plain sight during an annual procession by Christ Church Saint Laurence. *Courtesy of Christ Church St Laurence archives*

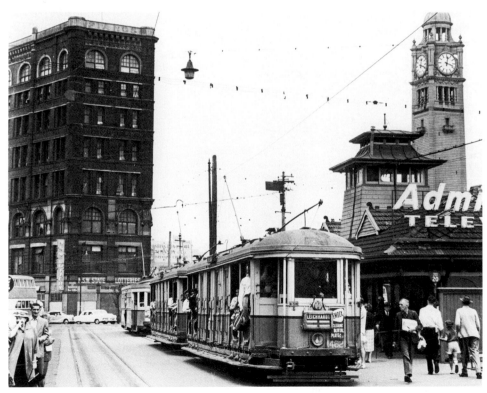

A typical Sydney toast-rack tram in Railway Square. Bee was famous for hitching rides on the running boards of moving trams. *Photo by Leon Manny courtesy of Sydney Tramways Museum Collection*

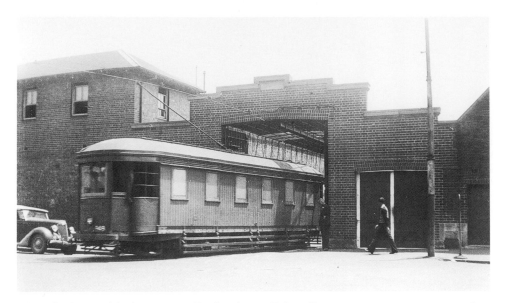

No. 948 Prison Tram entering Darlinghurst Police Station. *Photo by Norman Boxall courtesy of the Sydney Tramways Museum Collection*

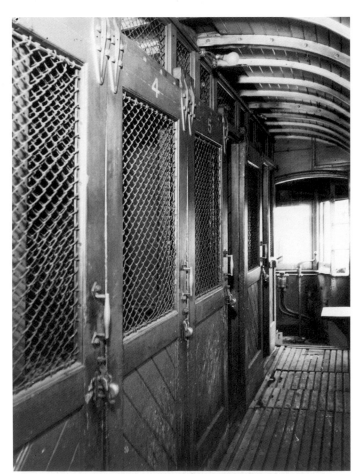

The interior of the No. 948 Prison Tram. Bee would have been familiar with the inside of this compartment. *Courtesy of Sydney Tramways Museum Collection*

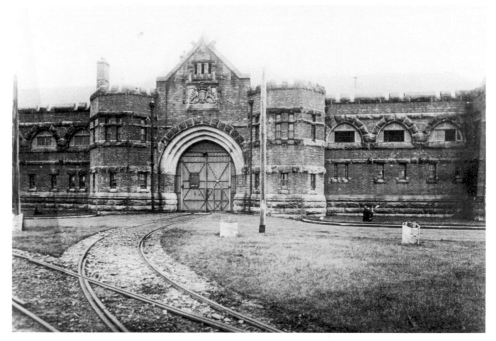

New South Wales Reformatory for Women, where Bee was sent on and off for thirty years. *Courtesy of Randwick City Library: A Social History Project*

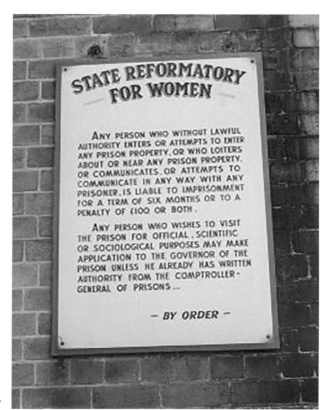

The sign at the gate
of the Reformatory.
*Courtesy of the State
Library of NSW*

These early articles from *Truth* (right) and *The Arrow* (below) mark the beginning of the media's fascination with Bee. *Trove*

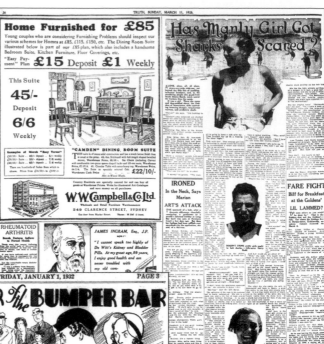

THE ARROW, FRIDAY, JANUARY 1, 1932.   PAGE 3

THE TERROR of the BUMPER BAR

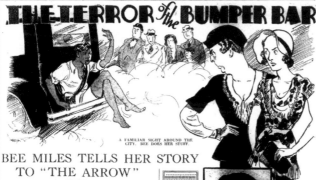

A FAMILIAR SIGHT AROUND THE CITY. BEE DOES HER STUFF.

BEE MILES TELLS HER STORY TO "THE ARROW"

She Rides Bikes and Bumper Bars

ASYLUM EXPERIENCES

A creature of moods, of wild impulses, a kind-hearted, well-educated, and cultured girl, but one whose pranks have earned her the reputation of being queer, is Bee Miles. She is known to thousands by sight because of her daily rides on bumper-bars and on her recently-acquired bike.

Here Bee tells her story, "The Arrow" revealing for the first time many intimate little details of the private life of the quaint, but attractive, personality.

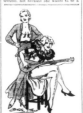

Here is a girl of splendid education who cares for convention, and lives a life of carefree nonchalance.

Callan Park

Despises Communism

"I heard that Tom makes love as if playing a beautiful harp."
"He does, if you play a harp with an axe."

— Jean Hull.

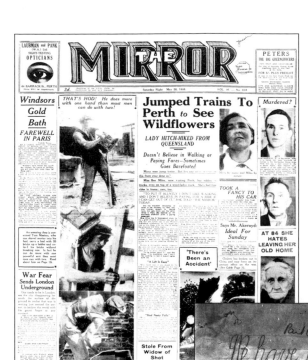

Bee on the front page of *The Mirror* after her arrival in Perth. The media coverage soon changed. *Trove*

Above: The opening page of Bee's unpublished manuscript 'Prelude to Freedom'. *MLMSS 1214, Frank Johnson Papers, Mitchell Library*

Left: The Publicist in 1938— William's name is conspicuously absent. *Author's collection*

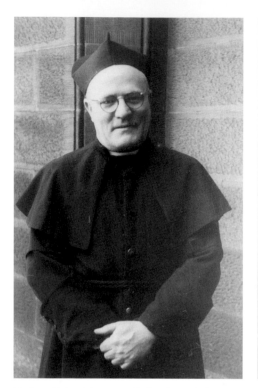

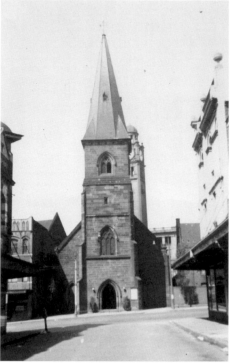

Father John Hope—defender of the faith and Bee. *Courtesy of Christ Church St Laurence Archives*

Christ Church St Laurence—Bee's refuge from police harassment and home for many years. *Courtesy of Christ Church St Laurence Archives*

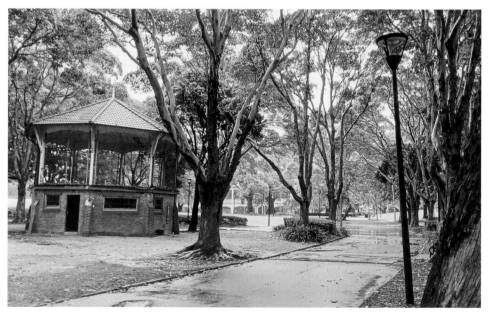

The bandstand in Belmore Park where Bee slept during the 1950s. *Courtesy of Arthur Branciad*

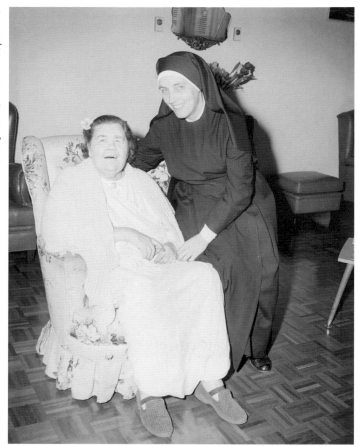

Bee with Mother Delphine at the Little Sisters of the Poor, 1969. *Photo by John Mulligan, courtesy of the John Mulligan Collection, National Library of Australia*

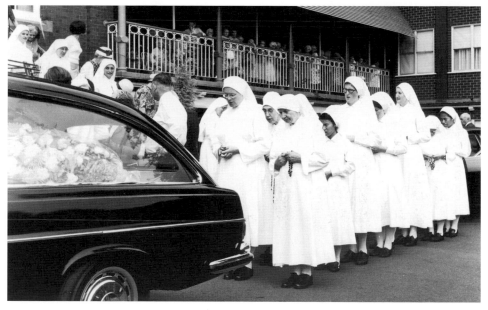

Nuns following Bee's coffin. *Courtesy of Sydney Archdiocesan Archives, Catholic Archdiocese of Sydney*

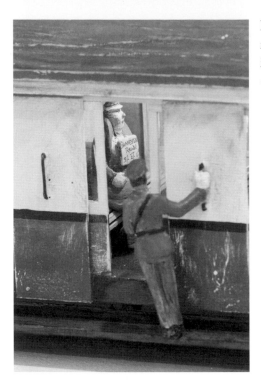

Peter Kingston's 2011 miniature model of Bee encountering a ticket inspector on a tram ride to Bondi.
Courtesy of the Peter Kingston Estate

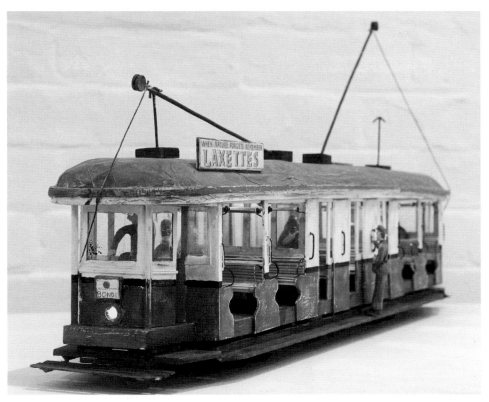

'Bee's last tram ride to Bondi', as imagined in model clay by Peter Kingston.
Courtesy of the Peter Kingston Estate

stay at the hospital had the opposite effect. She had 'a gorgeous time'; the matron 'was a darling'. They had long chats while she washed and ironed her dress. A local woman, hearing about her plans, came forward and paid her train fare to Mount Isa and she rode triumphantly to the station in an ambulance, grinning at the stationmaster who had originally handed her to the police. Reflecting on the experience, Bee turned her thoughts again to the familiar theme of human motivation and the malevolence of doctors:

> Dozens and dozens of men, women and many younger ones have told me and others that they would like to live my life; to ride on cars; to get lifts through the country; to do pretty well as they pleased. A doctor who obviously hated me . . . flatly denied that anyone would like to do as I do . . . he had made up his mind previous to examination to declare me insane . . . he told me that if he had his way he would keep me in Mental Hospital for good . . . I cried when he said that and told him he was a beast to try and frighten a girl. 'You're not a girl' said he spitefully, 'you're a woman'. Now a woman may call herself a girl while she looks like one; he probably made this remark because he felt he had not had as much fun in his youth as he would have liked.[13]

After being told by some miners on the train that Mount Isa was the prettiest town in Queensland, Bee arrived to find a maze of mines, tin shacks and dirt roads. But she was happy. She had made good progress and was now just under a thousand kilometres from her destination. Later that evening after Bee was evicted from the local hotel for playing a game of rummy in the lounge, she 'fell in' with two men: 'They lead me to a reservoir where we have the most glorious naked swim. I love swimming naked; it's a lovely feeling and in the dark . . . we have to feel our way through rushes.' She knew the men were after more than a swim, and she rebuffed them. They were 'womanly', and their suggestion of sex made her stomach heave. Having nowhere to go, she spent the rest of the night on the ground making good use of the mosquito net the kindly matron had given her in Longreach. The next day the police directed her to the CWA, who found her board and lodgings.

———

Bee was on the train heading back to Townsville. Most of the other passengers in her carriage were roaring drunk, but she was quiet, busy writing—trying to work out what had happened and put her thoughts into a rational order. She had planned to be away for at least a year and then bound for Europe. Instead, she was returning to Sydney after three months. It was at the Mount Isa boarding house that she first learned the bad news. A school had just been opened in Tennant Creek and the miners' kids wouldn't 'want any higher education'. Devastated, she sat on the steps of the police station. She had travelled nearly 3000 kilometres, battling for lifts, going without food, enduring the heat, being 'vagged', begging, foraging and even working, and 'all for nothing!' Her travel plans for Paris and London, the whole reason for this long, hard trip, were in tatters. On the advice of the CWA women, she boarded the train for Townsville, where they told her she might get some work. Depressed and tired, and in no mood for drunken conversations, she turned, as she had increasingly on this trip, to pondering about the irrational nature of human behaviour.

It seemed, she mused, that most people's social attitudes were shaped by their inhibitions, particularly around bodily functions. Why should the word 'lavatory' evoke feelings of disgust or shame, when it should be seen as a 'place of ease and comfort for the rectum'? Why should the average man feel shame when he hears the word 'breast', because he thinks that 'mating with a woman and feeling her bosoms is something to be ashamed of'? Why should a woman be assumed to be pathological because she also admires the aesthetic beauty of a woman's well-formed breast?

To have these reactions to mere words was 'stupid and unreasoning'. Yet her refusal to feel a sense of shame about them had been used as evidence of her mental instability when she was under observation at Mont Park Receiving House in Melbourne. She was still enraged by the experience.

Bee was finding things difficult in the train. It was crowded and noisy and she was continually forced to rebuff the attentions of a drunken passenger who had been trying to get her to drink a beer with him for hours. In frustration, she moved to the corridor to continue her 'pondering'. For all the foibles and inhibitions of the average man, there were times when she 'loved him very much', though it was purely platonic love. Some were, on rare occasions, 'delightful company'. As the train rolled on, she thought about those chance encounters with people who had given her brief moments of joy. The couple who gave her a lift, stopping for other strangers along the way until their car was full of laughter and tramps singing choruses. Or the man who suddenly took her hand in the city and leapt and bounded across the street in the middle of the traffic. The experience lasted only a moment, but she 'walked on air for the rest of the day'. But these moments of shared, uninhibited joy were rare and fleeting.

And what of life itself? Well, it wasn't worth much because it was too short and human beings were bound by their intellectual limitations. The average man believed that life was worth living because he was afraid to consider the alternative, but even so, he didn't get much pleasure out of life. Bee, on the other hand, who was unafraid to face the facts—that there was 'neither an afterlife nor a God'—knew life was meaningless but still obtained great pleasure from being alive, by living the way she chose. God was a human invention, conjured up because people were unable to 'face the horrors of life alone'.

By both design and necessity, she was alone—but was she really free? In typical rationalist style, she drew up a list under the heading, 'kinds of liberty':

1   Freedom of being able to do what one pleases
2   Freedom of speech
3   Freedom of being able to go where one pleases
4   Freedom of cosmopolitanism
5   Freedom from priggeries
6   Freedom of being out of debt
7   Freedom of being unmarried
8   Freedom of being heartwhole
9   Freedom of being under no obligation to anyone.[14]

She couldn't really do as she pleased, Bee conceded, because it always led to her arrest. She couldn't say what she wanted either. Despite her increasingly ambivalent views about her own sexual choices, she had been consumed by broader ideas about sexual freedom for many years and had read the work of sexologists such as Havelock Ellis and Norman Haire. She was even more convinced that there was a link between delayed sexual activity and mental illness, and that the age of consent was an arbitrary social construct, without any biological basis. This last claim was not an ambit one. Feminists and moral reformers had campaigned consistently since the nineteenth century to raise the legal age of consent, drawing equally on arguments about protection and control, particularly of young women. Bee argued that if the age of criminal responsibility was fourteen, then the age of consent should be the same. To be clear, here she was talking about sexual activity between young adults in the same age group, not between adults and under-aged minors. Nevertheless, it remained a controversial subject and Bee knew that if she discussed her beliefs on sexuality publicly, she risked being considered unstable and would possibly be returned to hospital. The experiences of William Chidley and his attempts at sex reform would have been in her thoughts as well. In the post-war period, particularly in the 1950s, Bee would return to the theme of sexual freedom and mental health with increasing conviction.

Love, as opposed to sex, was a topic that Bee found more difficult to analyse. She wanted to be in love but found it 'wearing'. Still on the train, and having finally repelled her drunken admirer, she started to list the attributes of her ideal man. He is someone with superior intelligence, who places no value on material possessions. He remains 'cool headed' even in a crisis, never losing his temper or raising his voice. These are qualities we might expect, and they would probably be a basic requirement for anyone in a relationship with Bee. But as the list continues, the ideal man begins to take on a different shape. He's a man who makes all her decisions for her, tells her how to dress and how to think. He doesn't 'give a rap' about her opinions but only wants her to listen to his. In other words, he wants to completely control her life. This man, she admits, would be 'the hardest man in the world for me to live with', but she might manage it provided she had a holiday from him every six months. While this description is at odds with what 21st-century readers might consider a healthy relationship, it would not have seemed so strange in the 1930s, when most aspects of women's lives were controlled and defined by male standards, including where they could work and how much they could earn. But how does this hyper-masculine archetype align with Bee's ideas about liberty and her earlier assertion that when freedom is lost, 'love dies'? Clearly it doesn't. The idea of Bee spending six minutes with someone so controlling is difficult to contemplate, let alone six months. Instead, her ideal man comes to rest in an idealised state—but remains the standard against which all the other men she encounters are measured and found to be 'womanly'. Their attempts at seduction make her physically nauseous, as her would-be seducers at the reservoir found out. But there is one exception to all these 'womanly men'—the writer H.L. Mencken.

Henry Louis Mencken (1880–1956) was an American journalist, essayist and social critic, who was both influential and controversial. His own influences ranged from Mark Twain to Ambrose Bierce to Frederick Nietzsche, whom he is credited with introducing to the American public. Mencken was a committed atheist who, like

Bee and her father, opposed organised religion in all its forms. As a satirist, he targeted middle-class complacency and social conformity. Human progress was not measured through material wealth and capitalism but through intellectual struggle—in the ability to seek the truth—to be an iconoclast. 'The iconoclast,' he wrote, 'proves enough when he proves by his blasphemy that this or that idol is defectively convincing—that at least one visitor to the shrine is left full of doubts.'[15] Under Mencken's satirical eye nothing was sacred, and he delighted in lampooning politicians and spiritualists in equal measure. Bee had been reading him since she was twenty and she was rarely without a copy of his *Chrestomathy*, an anthology of his essays and articles. It was this book that the psychiatrist had suggested was too 'heavy' for her in 1926. This would have only confirmed his value as a writer.

Along with her father William, Mencken had the most profound influence on Bee's intellectual and philosophical development and she continued to quote him for the rest of her life. He had one particular essay that she would have identified with strongly, entitled 'The Outlaw'. In it Mencken claimed that women's exclusion from society had given them a kind of anarchic freedom. 'In the midst of all the puerile repressions and inhibitions that hedge around them, they continue to show a gipsy and outlaw spirit. No normal woman ever gives a hoot for law if law happens to stand in the way of her private interest.' According to Mencken, 'The most civilised man is simply that man who has been most successful in caging and harnessing his honest and natural instincts.'[16] Bee would often say that Mencken was the only man she would consider marrying. But Mencken was already married to an American suffragette. He is her other ideal man, conveniently out of her reach. So she returned to her list and after analysing each of the remaining examples of freedom in the context of her current situation, it was apparent that, apart from being unmarried and having very few 'priggeries', she wasn't free at all. Liberty, she concluded, was like justice—non-existent, and love was just too hard.

When Bee arrived in Townsville, she sought the assistance of the Salvation Army but was soon 'in the bad books of the lady who runs its hostel'. From this point, the narrative drifts into unconnected sections, the writing, usually so neat and clear, becomes increasingly indecipherable. At the back there is a half-page scribbled fragment under the heading 'Dissertation on doctors and diverse subjects' that includes the following section:

> Over my trip from Townsville to Sydney down the coast I
> draw a discreet veil. One thing came of it. My knowledge of
> doctors, nurses and sisters of general hospitals was deepened.
> Hence the title for this part of the book. Only average men
> and women enter the professions of doctors and nurses.

Whatever occurred on the return leg of the journey clearly disturbed Bee. Was it another episode of mania or a particularly harsh arrest? Perhaps the collapse of her plans had affected her more deeply than she cared to admit, and she was unravelling. She never referred to the incident again. Like the episode where she kept removing patients' bandages, she built a wall of silence around it. She called the manuscript 'I Go on a Wild Goose Chase' and dedicated it to 'all those who helped me'. It was a rare acknowledgement that, despite the cardinal virtue of self-dependence, sometimes she had to depend on others. Before leaving Townsville, she had sent a letter to a book publisher:

> National Bank of A'asia
> Townsville
> Queensland
>
> Wednesday 4/12/35
>
> Dear Inky,
> What about the manuscript and introduction. Please write
> to me here and let me know about it. I am very worried.

When I left Sydney I went to Bathurst. Orange, Molong, Wellington, Dubbo, Nyngan, Bourke and Barringun which is on the Queensland border. Then to Cunnamulla in Q'Land, Charleville, Tambo, Blackhall, Barcaldine, Longreach, Winton, Cloncurry, Mt Isa and from there due east to here. Please write re the MS dear Inky

From Bee Miles.[17]

'Inky' was P.R. Stephensen, the proprietor of Stephensen & Co. book publishers. Most likely Bee was unaware that Inky Stephensen wasn't enjoying 'freedom from being in debt' either and that his equally grand schemes had fallen flat. Nor could she have known that once Stephensen entered her life, things would never be the same for either of them.

10

Blind Ambition

'If you are not for Australia—then who are you for?'

William Miles, radio broadcast, 1937

For any journalist reporting on the day, it would have been an unusual court case. Both parties were well acquainted with the courtroom and each other. On one side, seated behind his solicitor, was William John Miles, respected member of Sydney's commercial establishment, publisher and consummate litigant. On the other side, his daughter, Bee Miles. At 33 years of age, she was already a veteran of the judicial system, though usually as a defendant. But on this occasion, in July 1936, it was Bee who brought charges of unlawful assault against her father. And in a rare change she also had legal representation, Mr F.W. Cassidy, whom she sat behind.

Bee gave evidence first. She had gone to her father's office at 209A Elizabeth Street, to ask for a hawker's licence. She wanted to sell his newly launched political journal *The Publicist*. He asked her to leave but she refused. William became angry and began to 'punch her about the head and shoulders', and when she fell to the floor, he continued to strike her. By this time a policeman had arrived on the scene, one Constable Davis, and William hit Bee again as she lay prostrate on the ground, saying he would like to kill her.

In court the constable did not comment on this evidence, but said that Bee's two brothers, Arthur and John, who were managers at nearby Peapes & Co. in George Street, had arrived at their father's request and 'unceremoniously bundled her out of the office'. Bee said they carried her onto the street.

Under cross-examination by J.B. Sweeney, her father's solicitor, Bee acknowledged that she had legal action taken against her in multiple states as well as New Zealand and that she had been in several psychiatric hospitals. She admitted that she received a weekly allowance of £3 and 10 shillings from her father but denied the claim that she had gone to the office to seek his consent to travel to America.[1]

In his response William claimed that Bee was stronger than him and that if, in trying to get her to leave, he had hit her, 'it was an accident'. Referring to Bee's escape from Parramatta Mental Hospital with the help of *Smith's Weekly* nine years before, he told the court that his daughter had been 'quite sane until 1920'. He believed that she still had 'affection for me', adding 'I have some natural affection for her too.' In a final statement Bee declared, 'The only object of my life has not been to attract attention.' Since she had spent her entire career challenging notions of public order and propriety, this statement must have perplexed members of the court, as well as the attending journalists, who reported the proceedings in detail. At the magistrate's urging the parties reached a settlement and the charges were withdrawn. Bee agreed to stay away from her father's business.[2]

Ten months later, in August 1937, the parties found themselves in court again. The agreement, it seems, had been short-lived. This time it was William who initiated proceedings, charging his daughter with using insulting words against him and a second charge of offensive behaviour. Once again, the parties were seated behind their respective solicitors. Before proceedings began Mr Mack, acting for Bee, asked if her father might reconsider the charges. Both parties, he said, were respectable people, and a conviction would not be 'desirable'. After conferring with his client, Mr Sweeney, William's solicitor, replied in the negative. His client, he said, was tired of the defendant's 'everlasting annoyance'.

What had brought the two parties back to the courtroom in less than a year after their last, very public drama? According to William, his daughter had come to the Elizabeth Street office to remind him about her birthday money, in the form of a credit note at Farmer's department store. He had responded that he needed her address to complete the order. She refused to disclose it. A dispute followed, during which Bee called her father 'a poor old idiot' and a 'silly old fool'. William telephoned his sons to 'eject' Bee, as well as his solicitor and the police. The brothers dutifully appeared and threw their sister out, but she returned. Since her father had locked the door, she stood at the shop window pulling faces and moving 'her fingers about'. Under cross-examination, he said his daughter was 'insane'. Asked if he seriously meant that, he replied that she had been in eight mental hospitals.

Bee took the stand and said that she had been willing to provide her address but, before she had had a chance, her father had lost his temper and told her to leave. She had refused and sat in a chair while her father called her brothers. To keep up her spirits, she started to whistle, which appeared to enrage her father further, and he punched her and threw her to the floor. Her brothers arrived and ejected her, and she then returned and pulled faces at them through the glass and 'wiggled her fingers'.

The magistrate found the charges proved. The language was insulting and the behaviour offensive. He told Bee that she should have left the shop when asked and that both parties should 'avoid each other' in future. Bee was fined £5 and given a good behaviour bond for six months. She had come to collect her birthday money only to lose it in court fines. Her father declined to ask for damages. On leaving court she remarked to journalists, 'my father wants to put me away out of sight'.[3]

July 1936 was a challenging month for William Miles. Not only did he have to endure the public embarrassment of his private relationships being pored over by the newspapers yet again, but it was also an annoying distraction from the launch of a new project he had been planning meticulously for a long time. Over the last few years, he had been steadily winding back his business activities as a professional accountant and had closed his offices at Challis House. Initially, he didn't move far—just around the corner into Wingello House in Angel Place, where he sat in a kind of holding pattern while his new venture took shape. It was a plan, he confided to a colleague, that had had a long gestation. Unlike Bee, William had the means to travel overseas and did so frequently. He undertook four major international trips between 1924 and 1929, but it was after the 1926 tour, which included New York and Europe, that his plan to launch an 'Australia First' movement began to formulate. At first, he delayed putting any plans into action because he thought the mood in Sydney was 'unsuitable'. Whether this was a reference to the sustained industrial disputes that characterised the late 1920s, or his own personal battles with *Smith's Weekly*, is open to interpretation. But by 1933, he thought he saw a 'change of atmosphere, a change of psychological condition of the people likely to be sympathetic and receptive of new or contrary ideas'.[4]

The change of atmosphere was undeniable and had been building for well over a decade, as industrial unrest became more organised, and anti-Labor and anti-communist sentiment grew in response. Many wealthy industrialists and landowners had developed a siege mentality, which manifested itself in clandestine paramilitary groups such as the Old Guard and the King and Empire League as far back as 1917. These groups operated by forming cells, drawn predominantly from the ranks of former AIF men. The leadership, positioned in the exclusive, wealthy echelons of Sydney society with 'interlocking directorships' of banks and large companies, was secret. They relied equally on the loyalties of former AIF men, conservative rural associations and business networks—ready and willing to fight the perceived threat of communism against the Empire. Given William's wealth and commercial status, he should have been one of them— some of the leadership were his neighbours in Wahroonga. But at that stage William was aligned with their enemies, the Wobblies and Socialists. More importantly, their overt allegiance to the British Empire would have been anathema to him. During the 1920s, the Old Guard worked closely with the federal government, supplying men from their vast networks of returned soldiers to act as voluntary police during the seamen's strike under special legislation. The leadership of the Old Guard remained anonymous even though, by 1930, it had established an extensive network of cells and a membership of around 30,000 men. Many of its leaders went on to take up positions in the federal government's security services in later years.[5]

In 1931 Old Guard member Eric Campbell, a North Shore solicitor, broke away and formed a separate group he called the New Guard, a more overt organisation with a high public profile. The defection was almost immediate and New Guard membership swelled quickly. The tactics and behaviour of the New Guard were far more confrontational than anything the public had witnessed before. There were mass rallies at the Sydney Town Hall, with members brandishing fascist salutes. New Guardsmen were often armed, drilled regularly, stormed Labor party branch meetings and engaged in violent exchanges with communist groups. Their attraction to spectacle was exemplified by De Groot's performance at the Harbour Bridge opening. Campbell used radio broadcasts and newsletters to propagate their message—loyalty to King and Empire had to be protected from the threat of a Bolshevik revolution, embodied through the actions of the New South Wales Premier Jack Lang. Their level of alarm was so great that the leadership was said to have developed secret plans which involved sabotage and kidnapping. By the early 1930s membership of New and Old Guards was larger than both Commonwealth armed forces and the New South Wales police.[6] Campbell later claimed that he turned away hundreds of membership applications every week during the early 1930s.[7] In comparison, the Communist Party, the object of so much intense conservative paranoia, had around 4000 members nationally during the 1930s, though its membership rose to 23,000 during the mid-1940s after the Soviet Union entered the war. When Lang was famously dismissed by the governor, Sir Philip Game, the new premier told the people of New South Wales that they could go to sleep now—the country was safe.

These groups represented an extreme current of anti-democratic, anti-communist discontent that spread through the ranks of returned soldiers and into the broader community. Many commentators during the 1920s and early 1930s viewed the burgeoning power of fascist movements in Italy and Germany as cathartic alternatives to industrial unrest, high unemployment and modernist excess. Both the *Sydney Morning Herald* and *The Bulletin* published editorials extolling the virtues of a growing international trend towards fascism:

> The British Fascisti . . . is understood to be large and continually expanding. Its arrival in Australia is a good sign . . . Fascism is a method for organising a strong but inconspicuous counterforce, from which an army may be recruited to preserve civilisation should the existing forces fail.[8]

While the Australia First movement that William sought to establish, in its eventual form included fascist and National Socialist elements, its original vision was very different from the Old and New Guard organisations. William had no interest in the trappings of brash, paramilitary groups and their ostentatious behaviour, and his own idiosyncrasies would not lend themselves to any form of demagoguery. In 1935 his interests lay in setting the foundations for a movement towards an independent, secular nation state, where loyalties were not to the Empire, but to Australia First. It was an idea that he had developed during the anti-conscription campaigns twenty years earlier. Rather than mass rallies or secret cells, he had imagined the movement beginning with a series of small pressure groups of like-minded people that might grow to influence public and political opinion. His aim was to disrupt the status quo rather than maintain it. To set his plan in motion, he turned to the strategies he had used during an earlier, equally volatile political period. But this time, rather than relying on left-wing publications to circulate his ideas, he would start his own.

William launched the *Independent Sydney Secularist* in July 1935, writing the contents under a variety of pseudonyms. Its early issues were mainly concerned with restating the case for rationalism against religion, but over time they also revealed the dramatic swing in William's politics. He was now firmly anti-socialist and anti-communist and was against all political parties in the same way he was against all religions. There was another change as well.

In his early career William had been a stimulating and engaging writer. The contents of the *Secularist* seemed laboured and repetitive by comparison. It was never going to be the instrument to engender the sweeping change he sought. But then something happened that made him rethink his approach. He saw a new publication on a bookstand, *The Australian Mercury*, and read within its pages the first instalment of a three-part essay called 'The Foundations of Culture in Australia'. Its author was Percy Reginald Stephensen, known to most, including Bee, as 'Inky'.

———

Inky Stephensen was born in 1901 and grew up in Queensland. He attended university with Jack Lindsay and joined the newly formed Communist Party of Australia while still an undergraduate. He travelled to Oxford as a Rhodes scholar and continued with Communist Party activities until his scholarship was threatened.[9] After graduating he moved to London and joined Jack Lindsay and John Kirtley, who had relocated their Franfolico Press. Together they published many finely made first editions, including his own translation of

Nietzsche's *Antichrist*. Both Stephensen and Lindsay were moving in London literary circles though they were not always treated as equals by more established writers. Aldous Huxley famously included them as characters in his 1928 novel *Point Counter Point*, and the portrait was not flattering. They went on excursions with James Joyce and knew Norman Douglas (Bee's much-admired author of *South Wind*). Stephensen developed a relationship with D.H. Lawrence and published an edition of Lawrence's erotic paintings. When he visited Lawrence in France, the novelist complained that, after Stephensen had gone to bed, the walls shook for hours from the sound of his voice.[10] Stephensen was loud, brash and confident. He drank copiously and indulged in long sessions in the pub where he sketched out ambitious publishing ideas with a small group of expatriates including the Irish writer Liam O'Flaherty, a foundation member of the Irish Communist Party. Philip Lindsay, also in London at the same time, described Stephensen as a

> volatile communist with spasms of anarchism, during which he would drink noisily to the memory of the great Bakunin[11] . . . you heard him approaching the pub many, many minutes before he flung wide the door and entered bellowing for drinks all round. There would be backslapping, laughter, excitement . . . he stirred a pub to life.[12]

By the early 1930s Stephensen was facing financial hardship and tension was growing between him and Jack over Franfolico Press. At the urging of Jack's father Norman, Stephensen returned to Australia to establish the Endeavour Press, a new enterprise dedicated to publishing and promoting Australian writing. It was an ambitious project but proved to be ahead of its time. Publishing in Australia in the 1930s was a risky business. Most of the small presses failed and larger publishers, like Angus & Robertson, preferred to reprint popular international titles rather than local writers. Despite the backing of *The Bulletin*, the press failed, though not before it had republished Louis Stone's *Jonah* and a new book by Miles Franklin, who, encouraged by Stephensen and Lindsay, had also returned to Australia after being overseas for many years.

Undeterred, Stephensen, now committed to creating a dedicated home for uniquely Australian literature, launched his own company, P.R. Stephensen & Co. Most shareholders were prospective writers or their relatives, including Ruth and Victor White, whose young son Patrick had written a book of poetry Ruth was determined to see published. During the company's short life, Stephensen published the Henry Handel Richardson story *The Bath*, introduced Eleanor Dark's first novel *Prelude to Christopher* and was in the final stages of publishing a vast novel of over 200,000 words, from an unknown writer called Xavier Herbert, entitled *Capricornia*.[13] He also threw himself into Sydney's literary scene, joining the Fellowship of Australian Writers and hosting luncheons for the communist and anti-fascist journalist Egon Kisch[14] and the West Australian communist writer Katharine Susannah Prichard. He took over the editorship of Pakie's journal *Urge* and took part in regular public debates at the Club. This is probably where he met Bee and, she later claimed, developed a 'mild crush' on her.[15] Despite all this activity his own press was a financial failure, and the final blow was when a disgruntled printer melted down two tons of type that had been set for *Capricornia*.[16] By the time Stephensen launched his next enterprise, a magazine called the *Australian Mercury* in 1935, he was facing financial ruin. Ironically the first instalment of the essay it contained, 'The Foundations of Culture in Australia: An Essay Towards National Self Respect', earned him more praise and recognition than any of his former grand schemes.

In a broad and perceptive analysis, Stephensen's manifesto traced the history of Australian literature and intellectual life. In it he argued that the archetype of Australian culture—the bushman—had not only stultified and narrowed Australian literature but had aided in the destruction of the country's natural wealth in the service of the British Empire:

Millions of bales of wool, millions of slaughtered beef and mutton packed in ice, shiploads of gold, billions of bags of wheat have we ripped form our soil and dutifully sent home, home, home . . . Billions of trees destroyed and acres of grass eaten down to the roots . . . The Aboriginal human beings of the continent murdered, shot, poisoned; [sic] or enslaved, a human sacrifice to sheep brutally exploited, demoralised, the women raped, the children starved or taught about God in missions—in all this can we take any pride?

The essay's central argument was that a country was incomplete without a national literature. Until Australia could develop its own national voice and culture and wrote for itself rather than to meet the expectations of an English audience, it remained no more than a British colony. In defining nationalism, Stephensen sought to separate it from the aggressive expansionism of Italy and Germany, yet still utilised language and imagery common to pro-fascist ideology. Drawing upon notions of immortality and regeneration, he described national culture as a panacea for the decadence and fatalism of European modernist movements: 'The culture of a country is the essence of nationality, the permanent element in a nation. A nation is nothing but an extension of the individuals comprising it . . . When I am proud of my nationality, I am proud of myself.'[17] Ultimately, he argued, it was the artist, the writer and the painter, not the politician or the soldier who could help free the nation from the shackles of its colonial subsistence, through the creation of a national culture. The influences of Nietzschean and vitalist concepts are present in his arguments, as are the kernels of a pro-fascist ideology that would eventually lead to his demise.

No one had written about Australian culture like this before. The style was confident, the analysis sweeping and the prose persuasive. Many of the essay's arguments would be picked up again in the 1960s in a renewed push for an Australian cultural identity. The essay's publication engendered widespread praise from readers as varied as Billy Hughes, Mary Gilmore and Kenneth Slessor. It was a major influence on a young South Australian poet Rex Ingamells in the development of a new poetical movement—the Jindyworobaks. Although the issue sold well, it was too late for Stephensen, who was facing bankruptcy and had been hospitalised under the strain. But William read it and 'was delighted' by its content. He sought out Stephensen; though Bee would later claim that she brought them together. After some initial discussions William agreed to finance the final instalments of the essay and publish it as a book. The 2000 copies printed for the first edition sold out immediately. Stephensen, sensing the possibility of some financial security at last, drafted a plan for an Australia First party with a strong national defence system and almost total government control over banking and land allocation. William rejected the plan as too advanced and warned Stephensen about being too optimistic, as this only 'led to fits of depression'. 'Are we not entering another?' he asked.[18] By the time Bee was chasing 'dear Inky' from Townsville regarding her own manuscript and his promised introduction, Stephensen was already negotiating with her father to become his literary adviser for another publishing project. Despite the sometimes-terse negotiations, a kind of partnership was formed between these two men apparently so different—one shrewd, sardonic and pessimistic and the other, flamboyant, impetuous and, in his own words, 'Quixotic'. But they did share common traits—volatility, recklessness and an attraction to controversy.

In July 1936 William relocated to 209A Elizabeth Street in the T&G Building opposite Hyde Park—a luxurious and exclusive block of serviced apartments. The office, which included a bookshop, was the publishing headquarters of his new monthly publication *The Publicist*. Stephensen was paid a salary of £5 a week as his new literary adviser, which was raised to £10 later in the year. In its inaugural edition, *The Publicist* declared itself to be 'non-democratic, extremely anti-leftist . . . pro-Monarchical and pro-Rightest'. Stephensen the communist anarchist and William the socialist agitator had moved in a great pendulum swing across the political landscape. Attracted by the idea of an isolationist program under a corporate state, they would invest the same energy, enthusiasm and, in William's case, financial resources, into their current objective as they had done with their former allegiances. Their new direction was now fixed.

————

Each issue of *The Publicist* revolved around the repetitive themes of national independence, opposition to British economic domination and the nurturing of genuine Australian sentiment. There were other groups who had similar objectives, like the Australian Natives' Association (ANA), which advocated more Australian history in school curriculums, a greater use of Aboriginal rather than English placenames and the adoption of native flora and fauna in emblems and designs. But when the ANA invited a representative of *The Publicist* to join in their Australia Day celebrations, they received a curt response from William, who rejected Australia Day as 'a British celebration of the founding of a British colony'. He was also rankled by the fact that the ANA had supported conscription during the First World War, a theme he returned to repeatedly in his editorials, expressing concern that conscription might be reintroduced should a second war erupt in Europe.[19]

William wrote the editorials under the name John Benauster, while Stephensen wrote the column 'The Bunyip Critic' under his own name, and both wrote articles under a variety of other pseudonyms. Unlike his younger days on the Left, William never used his name in the publication. By now he had adult children and grandchildren and was no doubt anxious to protect their reputations, which had already been exposed publicly through their sister's growing notoriety. Along with Stephensen and William, there were several other regular contributors, mostly drawn from William's old anti-conscription and rationalist circles. There were no advertisements and William funded the entire publication. Its circulation was around 3000 copies per month.

To complement each issue and increase the publication's reach, Stephensen gave regular radio talks on 2KY and 2SM, where he argued for an increase in local industry not only to challenge British monopolies, but also to engender Australian development. For some Australians, emerging from the trauma of the Great Depression, and nervously watching the political eruptions in Europe, these words would have had resonance. They also held weekly discussion groups, at the nearby Shalimar Café, which they called the Yabber Group. Permanent invitations were issued to a broad cross-section of writers, artists and intellectuals, including Xavier Herbert, Dulcie Deamer, Tom Inglis Moore, Eleanor Dark, Lionel Lindsay, George Finey and Miles Franklin. Finey, Bee's friend and Pakie playmate, was strongly aligned with left-wing and workers' movements and may have attended out of curiosity at first, since Stephensen had been involved in left-wing activities up to that point. After the start of the Second World War, as *The Publicist*'s activities grew more and more controversial, government agents in a variety of unsuccessful guises began attending to take notes on any seditious behaviour.[20]

William was consumed with reigniting a campaign against conscription and dissuading Australia from entering any impending European conflicts. Stephensen, meanwhile, continued to harbour hopes that *The Publicist* might be a mechanism to establish his long-held ambition for a national publishing house. In 1937 he took a major step towards this goal by convincing William to finance the publication of Xavier Herbert's mammoth novel *Capricornia*, the draft of which had been sitting in a suitcase under Herbert's bed for five years, slowly being eaten away by insects. Finally, after years of struggle, revision, rejection and despair, this epic, sprawling uneven masterpiece came into being through Stephensen's urging and William's financial resources. It was entered and won the Common-wealth Sesquicentenary Literary Competition and the first edition sold out quickly. At last, it seemed they had backed a popular winner.

Meanwhile *The Publicist* articles continued to revolve around repeated themes of British dependence, weak leadership, falling populations, ecology and a lack of Australian identity. Their chosen subjects tapped into contemporary anxieties and conflated them with their own political agenda. Environmental reformers, feminists and eugenicists shared a common belief that Australia, with its large areas of open land and sunlight, could nurture a new, physically stronger breed to maintain its white population. This was exploited by *The Publicist*, which argued that this uniquely Australian type was in jeopardy of being emasculated by the decadent thrall of European culture. The country had become a place where cheap, imported culture and decadent commercialism overshadowed the 'spirit of the land'. Strong leadership was required to combat the declining and decadent population:

> We need here a Mahomet, a Hideyoshi, a Cromwell—or a Hitler—a man of harsh vitality, a born leader, a man of action, not one sicklied o'er with the pale cast of thought. Fanatics are needed, crude harsh men, not sweet and decorous men, to arouse us from the lethargy of decadence, softness and lies which threatens death to White Australia.[21]

Initially, this decadence was linked to communism and modernism, but increasingly it became part of a broader antisemitism by claiming that both British imperialism and Russian communism were part of a Jewish conspiracy. At the same time, speeches by Hitler began to be reprinted in their entirety, as well as a spirited defence of Japan's invasion of China. Although William and Stephensen both consistently denied they were fascists, there are elements of their rhetoric that have a close parallel to fascism. Fascist doctrine in the interwar period highlighted the need for a new order to regenerate a culture that had fallen into decadence. History was not a map of progress but a chart of decline into degeneration that needed an elite group to save the nation and lead it to rebirth and regeneration—a new order rising from the ashes. In most fascist ideologies, ultra-nationalism shares a co-dependency with racism, tapping into and exploiting common prejudices. When it developed its 'Fifty Points for Australia', its blueprint for a national restructure, *The Publicist* quite correctly claimed it was based on, and supported, the existing White Australia Policy, a policy that need strengthening to avoid a 'Semitic exodus' from Europe towards Australia as 'The Promised Land'. By continuing to link Jewish culture with communism and international conspiracies, *The Publicist* writers were able to promulgate racist propaganda while encouraging public anxiety about leftist threats. They not only subscribed to the infamous *Protocols of Zion*, but they also sold copies in *The Publicist* Bookshop.

Yet there was one topic that separated Australia First from similar contemporary pro-fascist and ultra-nationalist movements: its unequivocal support for Indigenous activism. For Stephensen, like Bee, this support was long-standing and while the origins of William's advocacy are unclear, he stepped up to the campaign with a vigour that recalled his former socialist zeal. In November 1937 *The Publicist* announced its full support for the newly formed Aboriginal Progressive Association (APA) headed by Jack Patten and William Ferguson, calling for an end to 'protection and government paternalism' that had all but 'exterminated' Aboriginal populations over the last 150 years. It urged the government to use the coming sesquicentenary celebrations to make some amends to the 'original owners of this land who have been so callously and cruelly dispossessed . . . They merely ask for citizenship. To withhold this is to perpetuate British atrocities in Australia . . . fair treatment of Aborigines puts white Australian decency to the test.'[22]

Stephensen and William had been introduced to Patten and Ferguson, both seasoned campaigners, through Michael Sawtell, a former Wobblie and anti-conscriptionist. Stephensen became secretary of the APA support group, the Aboriginal Citizenship Committee, and Patten and Ferguson were given space at *The Publicist* office to write and produce their monthly newspaper the *Abo Call*.

William funded the publication, along with posters, pamphlets, press releases and the APA Manifesto for the 1938 Aboriginal Day of Mourning and Protest. He even travelled out to the Aboriginal Reserve at La Perouse to speak at APA meetings—an arrestable offence.[23] Curiously, despite their public antagonism, he sometimes took Bee with him—or else she simply turned up. In 1938, in the build-up to the sesquicentenary, *The Publicist* support became more pronounced with every issue, William claiming that: 'From the first time of meeting until now, the whites have shown themselves to be inferior to Blacks. Only by guns and poison and greater numbers have they prevailed.'[24] Of all these activities, it was the financial resourcing of the *Abo Call* that was probably the most effective in spreading the work of the APA between Aboriginal communities and across geographical boundaries. At the same time, information about school segregation, inadequate housing and forced removals were fed back to the APA and reported regularly in the *Abo Call*, increasing awareness of shocking realities that were usually hidden from public view and providing evidence to strengthen the APA's political platform.[25]

While there was a genuine financial and philosophical commitment to the Aboriginal cause, there were also advantages for *The Publicist's* own political agenda. Support for the APA allowed William and Stephensen to deflect some of the growing opposition to their antisemitism. Those who chose to support external struggles by minorities, like the Jews in Europe, were accused of ignoring the exploitation suffered by Indigenous Australians in their own country. In promoting the APA, a further opportunity arose to criticise British injustice and the yoke of imperial submission.

But it is also important to note the competing voices around the Indigenous struggle in the 1930s, which had garnered support from diverse political, social and religious groups, often from opposing directions. Feminist organisations argued for an increase in protectionist legislation, particularly for women and children. Prominent anthropologists like Professor Elkin argued for a gradual 'uplift' to white society under the supervision of specialist anthropologists, while others argued for isolation to protect and preserve culture. The Communist Party of Australia and the trade unions supported a call for a separate republic and equal wages.[26] These competing voices, along with Australia First, caused division and disruption around and within the APA, which rejected absolutely a separation of Aboriginal people from the rest of the population, or a specialist role for anthropologists or protectors. In a radio interview with Stephensen in 1939 Patten made the APA's position clear: 'We don't want you to give us charity. We don't want you to study us as scientific curiosities. Give us education and equal opportunity, which is our birthright. Don't forget we are the real Australians.'[27]

In the lead-up to the Aboriginal Day of Mourning and Protest on 26 January 1938 at the Australian Hall, Stephensen wrote to the Australian Aborigines League—a white support group in Victoria—in response to their suggestion for a day of prayer. Stephensen told them their energy would be better spent sponsoring as many Aboriginal delegates as possible to attend the Sydney meeting. Over the last 150 years, he argued, Christians had nearly prayed Aboriginal people to extinction.[28]

But equally, Ferguson and Pearl Gibbs, a prominent Indigenous activist, clashed with what they saw as William's paternalistic attitude, while the Communist Party became increasingly vehement in its attacks on Australia First. Patten and Ferguson split in 1938 and formed two separate APAs. The movement eventually reunited but it lost support as the war moved into the forefront of national concerns. Patten enlisted and was sent overseas—the very thing that William and Stephensen had feared—but he maintained a close relationship with William and corresponded with him often. Whatever its motives, Australia First remains one of the few organisations of the period to provide practical resources for the Indigenous struggle to be articulated by Indigenous people, rather than on their behalf.

Stephensen's early *Bunyip* contributions had covered a variety of topics and usually included well-crafted reviews of new Australian books—a welcome contrast to William's ponderous prose. Increasingly though, Stephensen's contributions became defensive and repetitive railings against commercial publishing, modernity and feminism, which were all linked in his view. Critics of *The Publicist*, who were increasing in number, had their letters published, only to be followed by at times shrill and disproportionally lengthy responses from the editorial team. When Peter Lindsay, Lionel's son, wrote a letter complaining about Stephensen's attacks on Australian booksellers, William responded: 'I wonder if any Lindsay from your families will ever favour Australia First.'[29] Similarly, when Ida Leeson, the Mitchell Library's senior librarian and regular Pakie's member, wrote a short one-page response to Stephensen's public criticism of the library's failure to produce a catalogue of Australian books, Stephensen's reply went on for seven pages.

The antisemitism in *The Publicist* was matched by its anti-feminism and linked to the ever-pervasive threat of decadence.[30] Consciously manipulating contemporary fears and prejudices against women's employment as a threat to the traditional status of male breadwinners and incorporating it into a nostalgia for a past golden age, Stephensen wrote:

> Gone are the robust pioneer days ... Australia's females are now become vessels, not so much of maternity but of modernity ... Post-war hysteria, post-war boom, post-war emancipation of women, the drift from domesticity, the drift to decadence, to office jobs, to 'equality with men'.[31]

Miles Franklin, who continued to support Stephensen on a personal level and attended the Yabber Club meetings, wisely refused to submit any articles. Despite her own nationalism and growing anti-semitism, she had witnessed the anti-feminism in its pages and could not bring herself to be associated with it. She had also been shouted down by William at the Yabber Club when she expressed a different opinion.[32]

After they had faced each other in court for the second time, Bee only made rare appearances at *The Publicist* office, but for William there were continual reminders of her presence. Sydney was still a small city and many people knew who Bee Miles' father was. Taxi drivers would occasionally attempt to obtain a fare they claimed Bee had refused to pay, but William would angrily refuse them, stating they should have known better than to accept her as a passenger in the first place. The Commonwealth Savings Bank at Martin Place, where her allowance was paid, occasionally allowed her an overdraft, which William also paid. But when Bee would come to the office seeking additional funds, things became explosive. Jack Lockyer, Stephensen's stepson, worked in the office and was a witness to their volatile meetings. 'She would come into the shop and demand extra money and he'd say "Get out"; his face would become very red and they would have a shouting match. On one occasion he said to the typist, "Call the police!". Sure enough, the police came and dragged her out kicking and screaming.' Jack also noted that on these occasions Bee would appear in bare feet, attired in 'a dirty old dress with a torn sweater' (perhaps as a way of illustrating her poverty to her father). But when she went to visit Jack's mother Winifred, whom she liked, 'she was in the latest fashion dress with stockings, lipstick, powder, speaking very nicely and quietly'.[33]

William had repeatedly stated that the aim of Australia First was 'limited to arousing in Australians a positive feeling of distinctive Australian patriotism' and not to 'found a new political party'.[34] Yet by 1938 articles began to appear calling for volunteers to form an Australia First Party. The platform included informal voting, opposition to conscription, Australian-born governors, no overseas military campaigns, elimination of women of childbearing age from the workforce, compulsory labour training and employment of all youths, and the inclusion of Australian history, literature and art in school curricula. The response was lukewarm and after war broke out in 1939, the plan was quietly shelved by William, who planned to relaunch it after the conflict was over.

And so it continued, issue after issue—railing against the British, praising the military aggression of Japan and Germany and trying to lay the foundations for a new Australian Order, looking increasingly totalitarian in each of its iterations. *The Publicist* ran from 1936 to 1942. Reading its pages from a distance of 89 years, it is almost unfathomable how the publication continued for so long, particularly after Australia entered the war. Stephensen's biographer, Craig Munro, has argued that if a Labor government had come to power earlier, *The Publicist* would have been shut down.[35] Stephensen, ever the self-promoter, had been sending copies of his radio broadcasts to Prime Minister Lyons who wrote to him personally to congratulate him for 'the many admirable statements you have made on the need for developing in this country a national outlook and culture as a contribution to world welfare'.[36] Both Lyons and Menzies were early admirers of the loyalty and discipline National Socialism had engendered in German citizens, and in 1938 Japan was still considered an important trading partner.[37] Menzies had toured Germany in 1938 and was enthusiastic about what he saw, and Lyons famously chastised H.G. Wells during his 1939 Australian tour for publicly criticising the Nazi regime.[38]

But even as late as 1940, when there was no ambiguity about the extreme nature of *The Publicist*'s agenda, or Germany's intentions, the left-aligned H.V. Evatt, on the verge of resigning from the High Court and entering federal politics, invited Stephensen for a cordial discussion on the nation's state of affairs.[39] The architects of Australia First had a precise understanding of just how entrenched fears of shrinking and vulnerable white population were in Australia's democratic 'social laboratory'. Their antisemitic and anti-feminist policies, though voiced at an increasingly hysterical pitch, were firmly grounded in contemporary political thought and quite often in legislation. In the meantime, the Communist Party was declared illegal under the National Security regulations and several communist publications banned. But issues of *The Publicist* could still be bought in local newsagencies across the country.

This laissez-faire attitude did not mean that its publisher escaped scrutiny from both the military and federal security services. Initially, this was in response to complaints from the Communist Party and concerned individuals, who were becoming increasingly outraged by William's editorials and Stephensen's personal attacks on his critics. When a waitress at the Shalimar Café complained about some of the discussions she overheard during the Yabber Club meetings, representatives of the Commonwealth Investigations Branch (IB) visited William. His response was to angrily evict them and threaten them with legal action. The report on the incident noted that shutting down a small publication would 'do more harm than good' and that it was more antisemitic than subversive to the 'British Empire'.[40] A senior officer in the Eastern Command said that William was well known to him personally and no further action was taken. There were also consistent rumours that *The Publicist* activities were funded by the German government—a note had been pinned on *The Publicist* office's door which read 'German spy paid by Goebbels'.[41] Using the *National Security Act* (1939) the IB requested William's financial records from the National Bank of Australasia, which confirmed the far more prosaic reality that William had been running the operation as a tax loss. It was the Australian, rather than the German, government that was subsidising their propaganda. Along with details of William's income and investments, the bank also provided its own assessment of his character. It described him as 'shrewd in personal business but considered very eccentric', with the curious statement that he 'would be easy prey to a man with fixed ideas'. This confirmed the IB's suspicions that Stephensen, for whom they could find no bank account at all, was 'the brains of the operation'. But then again, they also thought he was married to Bee.[42] They concluded that William was a 'crank and a rationalist' but 'would not injure the well-being of Australia and appears to us to be wholly in favour of Great Britain'.[43] In this and so many other things, they were wide of the mark.

11

Fame and Infamy

'Wanted 500,000 young Australians, must be physically fit,
perfect in wind and limb for use in Europe as soil fertilisers.
Apply, stating nitrate content of body, to No.10 Downing
Street, England.'

P.R. Stephensen, *The Publicist*, July 1936, p. 4

Manly beach was hot and crowded. The newspapers estimated that there were more than 10,000 people gathered on that last Saturday of summer in 1938. They had come to watch teams from across Australia and New Zealand compete in the Inter Dominion and Interstate Surf Carnival. Spectators were treated to a wide range of competitive heats and march pasts, as surf teams vied for the championship. The surf was uncharacteristically calm.

But not so the lifesavers, and in particular the beach inspector, Albert Henry Owen, whose attention was focused, not on the huge crowd or the competing teams, but on a single female who had swum into an area cordoned off for the carnival. Like most of the crowd, he knew this woman, or knew of her. Hadn't she been banned from Manly by the mayor for swimming beyond the flags with a knife strapped to her thigh a decade before? Yet here she was again, ignoring the summons to return to shore and instead swimming out further and further until she hit a deep channel and was carried out 150 metres. She then swam another 230 metres to a line of buoys.

By now the crowd's attention also began to move from the competition to what looked like a very unusual rescue attempt happening offshore. With the now-furious inspector barking instructions through a loudspeaker, not one but two boats full of lifesavers rowed out to rescue the swimmer, but each time they managed to get her in the boat, she dived back into the sea. On the last attempt, a member of the crew jumped into the water to 'help' her and the boat was swamped. In the ensuing chaos, another crew member collided with the boat and had to be taken to hospital to have a gash above his eye stitched. Finally, the inspector himself swam out, and with the assistance of yet another lifesaver, escorted the woman back to shore.

A constable was waiting on the beach. At first the woman refused to give her name but eventually identified herself as Bee Miles of Bourke Street, Darlinghurst. Then she promptly turned around and went back into the water.

Incensed, the inspector followed her out. By now the whole crowd was watching as the two stood facing each other waist deep in the surf.

'Don't put your hands on me,' Bee commanded in her best Abbotsleigh voice.

Unwisely, as it turned out, Owen ignored her, and so, with a crowd of 10,000 looking on, she slapped him across the face and tried to pull his hair.

'All this happened in full view of thousands of people,' he later told the court. 'The behaviour was very offensive to me . . . it made me feel ridiculous.' No doubt he felt even more ridiculous when the story was circulated in newspapers from Melbourne to Auckland.

Bee, whom the papers described as a 24-year-old student (she was actually 36), argued that she hated people touching her in the water and that 'when I hit him it was a reaction to my fright', adding that she thought her head was being pushed under water. The magistrate was unimpressed by this argument, as well as the one her lawyer, Mr Meagher, put forward that, because the incident had happened at sea, the court had no jurisdiction. Bee was fined £1. 'Anyone would think I was undressing on the beach there was so much fuss,' she commented.[1]

———

At some stage in 1937, after repeated urging from Bee, Inky Stephensen wrote the long-promised foreword to one of her manuscripts. Modestly giving himself the title, 'eminent Australian literary critic', Stephensen introduced Bee as a 'skilled pianist and botanist', from an 'excellent family', who was beautiful, despite her tendency towards 'bizarre attire'. Though the manuscript was about Bee's 'wanderings', Stephensen also mentioned her battles with transport authorities and her questionable diagnoses and frequent hospitalisations, from which she was discharged as 'hopelessly sane or as indescribably mad' and concluded that Bee was 'a practising Individualist . . . in a community becoming increasingly standardised'. He concluded, 'The community will defeat this Egotist I have no doubt, but more's the pity.'[2] He could have been writing about himself.

The foreword was submitted to the publisher Frank Johnson sometime in the 1930s, but it was not attached to either of Bee's travel manuscripts. Instead, it was submitted with 'Prelude to Freedom', the retitled memoir of her 1920s committal and escape from psychiatric care. It is unlikely that Stephensen knew of her intentions. By 1937 he had firmly identified himself with William's Australia First vision and, apart from the occasional income derived from a writing partnership with Frank Clune, he was totally dependent on his stipend from *The Publicist*. If he thought he was writing the introduction to a book that accused his employer of predatory and violent behaviour towards his own daughter, it is highly unlikely he would have agreed, let alone have included the phrase,

'I believe every word in this present book is true'. He was aware of William's litigious tendencies and would have known about the very public schism with his daughter. After all, their spectacular fights had happened in *The Publicist* office. This then raises the question of why Bee placed the two documents together. Was it resentment against her father, who by then had taken her to court and made it clear publicly and categorically that he wanted to sever their relationship, or was she using Stephensen's literary reputation, still strong in 1937, as a way of securing publication? Though she was still no closer to publication, she still believed in the manuscript's worth. She had even tried to sell it to the highest bidder, possibly in a moment of financial desperation, a few years earlier.[3]

By 1939 she may have regretted asking Stephensen to write the foreword. His reputation was in serious decline. Many of his former supporters had grown increasingly alarmed by the changes they saw in their old Nietzschean-Bakuninite friend. In a bitter letter to fine book publisher John Kirtley,[4] who had been attending Yabber Club meetings and corresponding regularly with William, he complained that 'the entire constellation of Australian writers who wooed me so sedulously when I was a book-publisher were conspicuous by their absence when I started a real propaganda of unequivocating Australian Nationalism'.[5] The point Stephensen could not, or would not, acknowledge was that by the late 1930s the majority of intellectuals who had flirted with and even condoned National Socialism earlier in the decade had, in the face of undeniable Nazi extremism, withdrawn their support. Those already on the Left were even more galvanised into anti-fascist resistance. Xavier Herbert had long, rambling conversations with Stephensen over most of the 1930s about the genius loci—the spirit of the land—but eventually broke with him in a bitter dispute over *The Publicist*'s antisemitism. Herbert's wife, Sadie, was Jewish. On the other hand, the cultural and political renaissance offered by *The Publicist* also attracted support, despite the extreme nature of some of its statements. In 1938 Clem Christensen, who would later launched the literary journal *Meanjin*, had written to *The Publicist* regarding the formation of Australia First groups, saying he would be ready to join a group and assist if one was set up in Brisbane, but it never came to anything. Over the next few years Christensen grew increasingly disenchanted with Stephensen's growing jingoism and William's chauvinism.[6] But as late as 1942 Professor Elkin, the eminent and influential anthropologist, stated he would subscribe to *The Publicist* because its work would be of 'great value' in the future.[7] Though he was raised an Anglican, Elkin's father had been a Jewish rabbi in New Zealand. Security reports in 1940 noted that members of the Yabber Club (possibly William) had claimed that the Catholic Archbishop of Brisbane, who obtained copies of *The Publicist* indirectly, 'wholly approves of its policy as regards the Jewish question'.[8]

The 'Jewish question' received special attention from William in a 1940 editorial, when he stated that there could be no answer to the 'Jewish problem . . . while a Jew lives'.[9]

If this appallingly sinister statement, designed to provoke, created a backlash in the community, it did not result in any action from the Government. Investigation Branch reports noted that the 'only real objection is anti-Jewish attitude . . . I cannot help feeling that Miles is more eccentric than dangerous . . . Most complaints coming from the Jewish community. No doubting his loyalty to Australia.'[10] In fact, it was William who wrote to Police Commissioner MacKay complaining that for months the rabbi of the nearby synagogue in Elizabeth Street would pass by the office and shout 'how's Hitler . . . you dirty Nazi spy'.[11] No action was taken, but the police file noted that William was Bee's father.[12] Bruce Muirden, who wrote an otherwise perceptive study of the Australia First phenomenon, described William's attitude as a 'mild but persistent anti-Semitism'.[13] It's clear that it was much more than that. It was an obsession that had begun with religious opposition and evolved into racial vilification. Unfortunately, in Stephensen, he found a fellow traveller and they fed each other's irrational and outrageous conspiracies.

Bee was facing her own challenges. After her spectacular appearance at the Manly carnival, she headed for the other side of country, landing in Perth after fourteen days, which, she announced to the press, was a new record. The trip had included an arrest in Port Augusta, where she was gaoled for several days. Initially she received a positive reception by Perth journalists to whom she gave numerous interviews. The *Daily News* gave her lengthy coverage, introducing her to their readers as an exotic vagabond. 'She has no home . . . no husband and family. She looks twenty-five. She smokes. She doesn't mind being rather hungry when she can smoke. She loves pretty clothes but can't afford them and she'd rather read. She has slept out in the open often. She loves grand opera. Wagner is rather good.'[14] The *Mirror* ran a front-page interview, accompanied by a photo of a demure-looking Bee. Readers were treated to a detailed discussion of 'train jumping as a profession'. It was a dangerous occupation, she told journalists and firsthand knowledge was essential. 'From a platform it's simple, but it takes pluck to pull yourself up from the ground into a truck or van on a cold pitch black night.' She was 'a conscientious objector' when it came to paying train fares, she said.[15] Other articles covered her views on the importance of art, music and living a simple, happy life.

Stories of her epic trip appeared in Sydney papers as well. This time the reason she gave for travel was to study wildflowers in Geraldton, but she seemed to have remained in Perth for several months. She was staying in a boarding house in Frances Street run by yet another 'motherly' woman. By August she was beginning to be known locally as the 'woman with the sun visor' and the nature of the reporting started to change. In a small, provincial city like Perth, with a population of 280,000, and with such strong media interest, Bee's presence would have created both curiosity and controversy—and guaranteed police scrutiny. Inevitably this led to her arrest, after she climbed into the passenger seat of a car in the city centre and issued a command to 'drive on!' Unfortunately, the constable who had been following her also got into the car and they all drove on to the police station. She was arrested for refusing to give her name. In the Magistrates Court of Western Australia, the 'conscientious objector' defended her actions: 'Nobody can honestly say I'm mad. Yesterday I was simply trying to catch a bus . . . What is so odd about it? I do bail people up in cars, it is an economic way of travelling if you haven't the money wherewith to pay fares.'

Informing her that he was not in a position to 'discuss ethics', the magistrate referred Bee for observation. She was on the front page of the *Mirror* again, but this time the story was rather less celebratory. The article was picked up and versions were circulated across the country, under the headline 'Mental Test for Hitchhiker', reporters noting both her cultured voice and bare feet as she stood in the dock.[16] It's unclear whether she was released or extradited back to Sydney. She never referred to the experience again, but whatever the outcome, like Melbourne, the city of Perth was not as accommodating as she might have hoped. Meanwhile, Kenneth Slessor, describing her as 'the distinguished Australian traveller and female-explorer', awarded her 'the order of the golden hoof' in his *Smith's Weekly* column.[17]

But Bee's return to Sydney was not successful either. By 1939 she was back in court again, but this time it was under her own volition. She had decided to sue Constable Clement Gold in the District Court for £100. In evidence before a jury, Bee said that she had been travelling in a milk lorry from the city to North Sydney. As she approached the toll-booth on the Sydney Harbour Bridge, Constable Gold appeared and informed her he had a warrant for her arrest. He then forcibly removed her from the vehicle and detained her for several hours in the collector's box. Rather than producing any evidence of charges, he rang three different stations in search of any outstanding warrants. He eventually released her without charge. Outraged by Gold's overzealous policing, Bee returned the next day and took down his number. His actions, she claimed, had caused her to suffer 'great pain in body and mind . . . [she] was exposed and injured by her credit and circumstances and prevented from going about her business'. She told the court, 'It is frightful to lose your liberty.'

On the witness stand, Constable Gold's barrister challenged her claim that his client had damaged her reputation. Under his questioning, Bee admitted that she had been in trouble for swimming out beyond the buoys at the beach, for smoking on the Cenotaph, for stopping a train and for hitting a man. She gave a slight smile as he reeled off the offences. 'In fact,' he said, 'you are the famous Miss Miles who hops on and off trains and trams and scales everywhere.'

'Putting it as nicely as I can,' the barrister said, 'will you admit you're eccentric?' In a sudden departure from her usual courtroom bravado, Bee began to sob. The barrister had hit a nerve. Eventually she responded, 'I suppose some people would call me an oddity', and apologised to the court for breaking down. The jury found for Constable Gold, who had denied all charges. Observers in court had been used to seeing Bee defiant, humorous or indifferent, but always composed. She had never broken down in public before. The entire experience had been humiliating.[18] Like the unfortunate Manly beach inspector, the results of the case were reported throughout the country and as far as New Zealand.

It wasn't the only courtroom defeat in 1939. In a libel case that same year Stephensen had sued the Communist Party's newspaper, the *Worker*, for £5000 in damages for libel, after they published an article accusing him and *The Publicist* of being propagandists for German and Japanese 'Warlords'. He and William were found guilty of contempt in the lead-up to the hearing and had to pay damages. When the libel case was finally heard, the jury found in favour of Stephensen but awarded him a farthing (a quarter of a penny).[19]

From April 1940 William was required to submit each issue of *The Publicist* to the censor. He was happy to comply, seeing any of the content that was passed by the censor as a type of official endorsement. While the censor did pass each issue, some of the more aggressive antisemetic articles were removed. From a 21st-century perspective, why it took so long beggars belief. But in the 1930s antisemitism was overt and could be found across the spectrum of public and private debate, from political rhetoric to the more refined conversations of the Royal Sydney Golf Club.[20] Once censorship started, William immediately shut down his other publication, the *Independent Sydney Secularist*. Security officers seemed much more interested in that small, intermittent, four-page circular than anything else William was publishing, but not so much for its racist content. They were convinced that it was linked to the Rationalist Association and communism—even though William had broken publicly with the latter years before.

Although Stephensen and his employer had dreaded the idea of another war, they now saw it as an opportunity for renewal. They thought that the allied forces faced certain defeat against the might of German military aggression, that Japan would replace a crumbling British Empire in the East and that, from the ashes of destruction, a new Australia would rise. They were in effect, waiting for the revolution—a revolution that would produce an independent Australian identity. It had been the revolutionary aspects of fascism, along with its sustained focus on culture and place, that initially offered significant appeal for Stephensen. In its early stages many intellectuals were attracted to fascism because of its emphasis on aesthetic values and its promise to 'restore culture as well as society'. Perhaps, equally as important, it was a movement that appeared—at least initially—to allocate a special role for intellectuals 'as guardians of social values'.[21] Ultimately this is the role that Stephensen began to carve out for himself and the Australia First Movement. *The Publicist* had produced an 'idea of Australia', but it needed further refinement, and this was the role of the poet. An ideal situation would be a combination of 'poetics and political', which he claimed had occurred in Ireland.[22]

William was a far more seasoned and cynical campaigner, and was more ambivalent about the future. The fact that war had been declared left him depressed and deeply concerned, because he believed that Britain was headed for defeat. As devastating as this was, however, it could lead to a kind of catharsis because it would 'force them [Australians] to put their own interests first through the instinct of self-preservation'.[23] But before that happened, 'there could be a minor revolution'. 'These forties,' he wrote, 'will scream as well as roar, and blood will not be shed abroad early. The magnitude of the error is so enormous that very little of the Empire will escape the trouble . . . but I am too worried to labour the subject—it is all too upsetting.'[24] Neither Stephensen nor William believed that Japan would attack Australia but, once war was declared, they had started to tone down their rhetoric around Australians fighting overseas, acknowledging that Australia should support Britain against Germany, though only on a voluntary basis. There were no concessions around conscription as long as William was still in charge of the contents.

But by 1941 William's grip on control was increasingly tenuous. After years of battling a heart condition, he had developed gangrene in one leg and was in excruciating pain. He still managed the publication from his sick bed and was planning to shut it down for the duration of the war. Instead, an agreement was reached to sell *The Publicist* to Stephensen and two partners for £5. He had already changed his will in 1940, dividing his estate valued at nearly £50,000 unevenly between his children. The bulk of the estate comprised of shares in Peapes & Co.—which had continued to trade profitably in the 1930s, despite the Depression—along with a small number of shares in the New South Wales Crematorium Co., which managed the Rookwood Crematorium. Bee was to receive an annual payment of £360. The will also stipulated that, in the event of Bee outliving her siblings, she would never become an executor.[25] William had always believed that his recalcitrant daughter was a spendthrift, with no understanding of the value of money. He saw this as another sign of her 'insanity'. His will ensured that she would always have enough money to survive and avoid arrests for vagrancy, but it would be a frugal existence.

While William was moribund in his Gordon home, things around him were moving fast. The threat of a Japanese attack on Australia was foremost in the minds of the public and the new Labor government. Air-raid shelters had been constructed in the tunnels of St James and Town Hall stations, while the government strove to reassure an agitated public that there were no workers of 'foreign extraction' employed in munitions factories. Windows were boarded up and strips of paper were pasted across glass to prevent shattering. Onlookers watched with a sense of foreboding as the clock tower was removed from the GPO in Martin Place. Public transport stopped at midnight and car headlights were permanently dimmed.

Ironically these heightened security measures coincided with an increased sense of freedom for women. There was a shortage of manpower and, for the first time, women were actively conscripted into the male roles that they had been previously denied access to, which meant they were also receiving a male wage. In most cases this doubled the usual women's wage. The government made it clear that this was a temporary measure. For other women, who remained in traditionally female occupations, their wages remained the same. With a constant influx of soldiers, both Australian and later American, into cities and towns, demands for services of all kinds increased dramatically. Women employed in service industries, such as hotels and cafes, worked long hours, as well as volunteering in the many canteens that were set up to cater for the armed forces. Over one million American soldiers were stationed in Australia during the war, mostly in 1942. Across urban and provincial centres, the pace of life accelerated, while at the same time, the social restrictions that had governed the lives of most women had loosened. It was a period that saw the rise of what military authorities called 'the amateur': women who were not prostitutes but were deemed to be sexually adventurous and publicly available. The threat they posed, apart from a perceived lowering of moral standards, was the spread of venereal disease and 'hundreds of women' were arrested in the company of soldiers for vagrancy, only to be released when it was found that they were actually employed.[26] The musician Merv Acheson, whom Bee knew well, described the mood in Sydney during a period when the future's uncertainty created a new urgency to find pleasure in the present:

> Sydney was a rip-roaring town during the war years. Every industry was working flat out, the Yanks were spending money like water, there was a flourishing black market, and the underworld was doing a roaring trade in everything from petrol coupons to nylons and liquor. In this atmosphere the entertainment industry boomed. Pubs which closed at 6 pm had very little liquor or so they said, but nightclub tables groaned beneath the weight of bottles . . . By law liquor was barred from dance halls, except on occasional ball nights when a special license had to be obtained. This left the nightclubs with an open slather as they were the only places providing liquor and entertainment. And they sprang up in their dozens.[27]

There is no evidence that Bee engaged in any activity that contributed to the war effort, either paid or voluntary. She wasn't conscripted into any wartime industries and, while she may have wanted to work, her notoriety and her behaviour would have precluded her, no matter how acute the shortages in manpower were. The only change was a slight decrease in her arrests. Perhaps the authorities were too busy policing the amateurs, who were estimated to be around 8000 in number at the height of the war.[28] According to the writer Betty Roland, who was a friend of Bernard Hesling and lived in Elizabeth Bay, close to Bee's home in Roslyn Gardens, 'the whole town throbbed with the pulse of overheated sex'.[29]

While Bee would have approved of the country's youth behaving 'a little recklessly', writers for *The Publicist* saw it as a further sign of democracy's decadence. In the lengthy tract 'Fifty Points for Australia', they had restated their call 'for women in the home' and 'against women in industry', even though women were now being mandated to fill wartime workforce vacancies.[30] But it was a woman's entry into their own enterprise that brought about a set of changes neither Stephensen nor William could have predicted. The fact that it was engendered by a feminist would have been bitterly ironic to both. In 1941, with William no longer in active control, Adela Pankhurst Walsh suddenly approached Stephensen with an ultimatum. Adela, the estranged daughter of the famous Pankhurst suffragette family, had been highly active in the Victorian Socialist Party and the Woman's Peace Army, and had been a co-campaigner with William in the anti-conscription campaigns. They had continued to enjoy a friendly relationship in the early 1920s, both contributing to socialist journals. Adela was a foundation member of the Communist Party of Australia, and William often teased her about her closet Catholicism.

By the 1930s Adela, like William and Stephensen, had made the journey across political lines, but they had landed in very different places. Adela, always in penurious circumstances, had founded and become chief organiser for the Australian Women's Guild of Empire (William called them 'Amazons of the British Garrison in Australia'). Her husband Tom, a former Wobblie and communist, had become a member of the New Guard. The guild, funded mainly by industrial groups, sought to nurture cooperation between workers and employers and discourage strike activity. This made Adela the subject of much derision when she visited factories to spread the guild's message. Alongside anti-union propaganda, the guild also promoted loyalty to Britain and British identity.[31] Both Adela and Tom had become strongly opposed to communism and were staunch admirers of Japanese culture and politics, as was *The Publicist*. The Walshes went on to cultivate a commercial relationship with the Japanese government that was their eventual undoing, when it funded their visit to Japan at the end of 1939.

As the war progressed and fears of a Japanese attack increased, Adela was dismissed from the guild she had founded, losing her much-needed regular income. She informed Stephensen that if he didn't work with her to form an Australia First Party, she would do it herself. In October 1941 a meeting was held in a North Sydney flat to establish the Australia First Movement (AFM). The eclectic nature of its executive is evidence of how quickly things had changed now that William was no longer in control. Stephensen was the president, while Adela and another former communist, Leslie Cahill, were paid organisers. Three former guild members, a truck driver and his wife, the owner of a shoe shop and the South Australian poet Ian Mudie made up the rest of the executive. Stephensen's 'Fifty Points' had been reduced to ten and modified to accommodate some of the wishes of the women on the executive. A series of weekly public meetings was announced, which commenced in November at the Australian Hall in Elizabeth Street, the site of the Aboriginal Day of Mourning and Protest that Stephensen had helped to organise and that William had supported financially. Around 100 people attended the first meeting on 5 November, including a group of noisy hecklers and some security officers.[32]

Novelist Miles Franklin, who had continued to support Stephensen, attended the meetings regularly. She was still attracted to Stephensen's ideas about nurturing Australian culture and subscribed to *The Publicist*, as did Mary Gilmore and Lionel Lindsay, but she never joined the AFM, nor, despite what is sometimes claimed, did she speak at any of the meetings. Her problem, as her biographer Jill Roe has noted, was that she remained supportive for too long and became tarnished by association in the process.[33] Bee was also present at some of the meetings and, on 13 November 1941, she joined the AFM, giving her address as 69 Roslyn Gardens, Elizabeth Bay. She also participated in the AFM's event to mark the anniversary of the Eureka Stockade, where she performed two poems, apparently to great dramatic effect.[34] Bee later insisted that her father never discussed *The Publicist* with her nor what he wrote for it, but she certainly would have read its contents and clearly still took an interest in his work.

Bee's own feelings about the war were more circumspect. She made no public comments, perhaps sensing that her father and Stephensen were creating enough public controversy on their own. In any case she had always been reluctant to speak about her family publicly. While there is no evidence of antisemitism in her own writing, she did become increasingly anti-British after the war, though her nationalism was always tempered by the realities of her personal situation. Still, it was a puzzling gesture for one who made a virtue of never joining any cause. Did she join in a futile attempt to please her father or out of perversity because he was no longer able to object to her presence? Perhaps she wanted to support her father in the same way she had during the First World War. But their relationship was now very different from the time when she had defended him in the school playground. Her father had cut the cord in a very public way during their court cases. Nevertheless, she joined the movement. Her brother John, from whom she was also estranged, joined as well.[35]

Throughout November and December and against a rising tide of public anxiety about Japan's march across the Pacific, the meetings continued, each one rowdier than the next. Left-wing protesters were joined by soldiers, and both were particularly antagonistic towards Adela. Public pressure was mounting to shut down the AFM, and Stephensen's name was mentioned in federal parliament. What the public didn't realise was that representatives from three different security groups had been monitoring Australia First activities for several years. They included the Commonwealth Investigations Branch, the Military Intelligence attached to the army, and the Military Police Intelligence, part of the New South Wales police under the auspices of Commissioner MacKay. Rather than sharing intelligence, they often held competing views, and their reports on the Yabber Club meetings, which each attended at different times, were conflicting. Throughout November agents from these various groups attended the AFM meetings, occasionally intervening when violence broke out, but not always. But by now the movement was already beginning to implode without external intervention. Adela was pushed out—her Japanese sympathies now recognised as a liability—and Cahill left to enlist. The broader membership never reached a hundred. The Investigations Branch, noting that the AFM was likely to collapse, had begun to reduce its surveillance but Military Police Intelligence was moving in the other direction. It approached Commissioner MacKay to close the movement down. He refused, claiming that was a Commonwealth responsibility. The public meetings continued, now moving to the Adyar Hall in Bligh Street, home to the Theosophical Society.[36]

The country entered 1942 with a heightened fear of imminent attack by Japan, but William was now beyond politics. Along with his failing physical health, the onset of another war had decimated him emotionally. In a rare acknowledgement of his own vulnerability and powerlessness, he wrote to John Kirtley admitting defeat:

> I feel that I shall be swept into a gutter and a grave, after an utterly futile attempt to help 'put things right'. I have never felt so completely useless, from sheer incapacity, to struggle successfully against community conditions, never before did I realise how little the individual is, relatively, with the community he lives in . . . Only in death will there be peace for me; I feel I really need peace and that in no other way could I get it, which is nearly the equivalent to throwing in the towel or kicking the bucket.[37]

Yet even in these last moments William summoned the energy to indulge his other abiding passion—gambling. For most of his life, apart from when he was travelling overseas, he attended regular race meetings at Randwick Racecourse, always betting on a losing system.[38] It might have been a way of reducing his tax burden but it also fed his appetite for risk.[39] (Bee also inherited a love of gambling though she bet on cars.) Now in the final days of his life, he ran a sweep on the exact hour of his death. He also wanted it known that, should he recant his atheism at any stage, it would have been because of the 'dispersal of his rational facility' due to 'the approaching dissolution of his brain tissues'. He never recanted.[40] William died on 10 January 1942. Bee had been allowed to visit him in his last days. She later said they had 'talked amicably . . . I felt such indescribable pity for him I couldn't bear malice'. For Bee, her father's sense of failure went beyond political struggle. 'He wanted my brothers and sisters to love him. They didn't love him. They were frightened of him, and they were frightened till the end of his life.' But was this actually the case? Certainly, he had been a harsh disciplinarian and demanded a great deal from his children intellectually. But Bee's sister Constance also remembered him as an indulgent father and a generous giver of gifts, and he had a very close relationship with his son John. Yet, according to Bee, 'he died a broken hearted, unhappy old man'.[41] There may have been another reason for his despair. He once told Jack Lockyer, Stephensen's stepson: "'I've had two great shocks in my life; one was ten years ago when I woke up in my bed and realised I'd had a stroke, I was shocked and horrified; the other occasion was when Bea recovered from [encephalitis lethargica] and I realised her mind had been affected." It was a tragedy to him because she was a really gifted person,' Lockyer added.[42]

William was given a rationalist service at the Rookwood Crematorium, where he had been a shareholder, on 11 January. Stephensen gave the valedictory address, which he later published. In deference to the family's wishes, the pseudonym John Benauster was used rather than William's real name.[43] On 14 January, the *Sydney Morning Herald* published a brief obituary of William John Miles, describing him as a leading Sydney accountant and founder of a political journal. On the same day *The Sun* published a page-two article on Bee, citing a magistrate's description of her as 'a public nuisance'. Charged with offensive behaviour for throwing a tram conductor's hat into a passing car, Bee claimed she had been defending herself against 'slander', after the conductor had made an offensive remark.[44]

On 19 February the country's worst fears were realised when Japanese bombs fell on the city of Darwin. With his usual appalling sense of timing, Stephensen held an AFM meeting that night at the Adyar Hall. Over a hundred waterside workers marched up from Sussex Street, where William had attended anti-conscription meetings two decades before. They were joined by other union representatives and soldiers, some carrying rotten eggs, while others held iron bars.[45] In a scene reminiscent of New Guard confrontations, they crashed the meeting. In the ensuing melee chairs were broken and plaster fell from the walls. While protestors stormed the stage, someone stole the membership book, containing the names and addresses of everyone who had joined. Stephensen was attacked—violently punched and kicked—yet rose bruised and bleeding, and continued to address the meeting, telling those present that it was 'All in the game. The Movement will go on undeterred by any Bolshevik bashers.'[46] The Military Police, present at the meeting, would prove him wrong.

The publicity that followed prevented the ever-ambitious Stephensen from hiring the Town Hall for his next meeting, so he booked a theatre in Manly instead. By now MacKay felt the need to personally intervene, as he had done with Bee years before (or so she claimed). MacKay had taken on and defeated many groups before this, including the New Guard, and took a similar approach with Stephensen. He summoned him to his office and asked him to cancel the meeting. Stephensen reluctantly agreed and told the executive he was putting a hold on the AFM as well.[47] But it was too late. On the other side of the country, action had already commenced that would ensure the AFM's demise, a public scandal and Stephensen's permanent fall from grace.

In a series of steps never really explained by any of the security agencies, Military Intelligence began an operation in Perth to investigate a local AFM group. The fact that no AFM group existed there was not a deterrent. They used a paid police agent, who had previously infiltrated communist groups, to approach four, possibly unhinged, *Publicist* subscribers. He told them he'd been sent by Adela to help set up an AFM branch. (Adela, by now, had already been ejected from the AFM.) With the agent's active participation, they developed a proclamation that included plans for potential sabotage (not dissimilar to the more extreme plans the New Guard had developed in the lead-up to Lang's dismissal). It also included 'absolute equality of the sexes'—an indication of how little they knew about the real AFM. But the third and most damaging item was the inclusion of collaboration with the Japanese. Armed with the 'Proclamation of the Australia First Government', Military Intelligence sent an urgent cable to Sydney.[48]

At four o'clock in the morning Stephensen, asleep and oblivious to any plans being hatched in Perth, was woken by four police acting for the army. He was taken to the cells at Central Station and then escorted to Liverpool Internment Camp, along with fourteen others associated with the AFM. He was not charged. Adela was eventually arrested and interned as well. They all thought it was a mistake and that they would be released quickly but in fact they were formally interned under National Security regulations, which allowed for indefinite detention without trial. Initially the government denied the internments had happened but gradually the truth emerged, and protests began to erupt. These grew louder when it was revealed that the Commonwealth Solicitor General, H.F.E. Whitlam (father of the future Labor prime minister), concluded that Stephensen had not committed any crimes under the *National Security Act* or any other Commonwealth Law.[49] At the same time it was becoming apparent that there was nothing to link the AFM with the Perth group, the Military Police Intelligence noting 'not one single piece of evidence has been obtained that the Movement here, or any one of its members, were party to or had any knowledge of the "Proclamation"'.[50]

While Dulcie Deamer was trying unsuccessfully to raise support for Stephensen from her fellow writers—he had offended far too many of them—assistance was coming from some unlikely sources.

Publications that Australia First had criticised so publicly in the past, like *The Bulletin*, the *Worker* and *Smith's Weekly* began to campaign for the internees to either be brought to trial or released.[51] Various churches also expressed their concern. Even members of Labor's own government began to complain and raise questions in federal parliament. Eventually some members were released on appeal, including the poet Harley Matthews. Matthews had fought in Gallipoli and was the model for the bronze soldier *The Spirit of the Anzac*, still housed in London's Imperial War Museum. He had a vineyard in Moorebank, outside Sydney, which had been the site for regular weekend bohemian gatherings in the 1920s, where an assortment of writers and artists would drink Matthews' wine and avoid a sometimes-inebriated pig.[52] Slessor had immortalised the vineyard in prose and in the poem 'Five Bells', when he and Joe Lynch had stumbled towards Matthews' place one night in a storm:

> Then I saw the road, I heard the thunder
> Tumble, and felt the talons of the rain
> The night we came to Moorebank in slab-dark,
> So dark you bore no body, had no face[53]

Matthews, like the majority of those interned, had peripheral involvement in Stephensen's and William's activities, and was later exonerated, but he was broken by the experience of internment and the public accusations of disloyalty. Eventually all the internees were released except one. Stephensen, obdurate as always, demanded a trial. None was forthcoming but Attorney-General Evatt finally agreed to an inquiry, where Stephensen was able to give testimony. By now he was very deaf in one ear and approached William's family for financial help to purchase a hearing aid. Through their lawyer, they declined to provide any assistance.[54] The Clyne Inquiry that followed cleared some internees, including Matthews, but maintained that Stephensen's internment was justified. It also provided a fascinated reading public with details of William's involvement in *The Publicist* by revealing the true identity of John Benauster.[55] Finally released on the day after Japan surrendered, Stephensen moved to rural Victoria and started a small press, which again came to nothing. He was bitter and isolated and told Miles Franklin he was finished, but not before underlining the value of his work:

> My distinctive contribution . . . was that I saw the necessity
> of linking Australian literature with political nationalism,
> the movement for political independence from Britain. As
> I got no support from Australian writers, I've retired from
> unequal combat. For eleven years, 1931–1942, I was a Don
> Quixote, then I was unhorsed.[56]

Ironically it was the contribution Stephensen had made to Australian literature before he linked it to politics that became his most enduring legacy. 'The Foundations of Culture in Australia' was to be resurrected by Donald Horne and other public intellectuals in the 1960s, and many of the initiatives he had called for in the 1930s, such as a national ballet, an opera house and chairs of Australian literature across Australian universities, would be realised, though not in his lifetime. Stephensen continued his writing partnership with Clune and produced several successful books. He also received considerable support from book collector and fine book publisher Walter Stone, while Dulcie Deamer and Miles Franklin remained in contact. Younger writers, including the historian Manning Clark, made pilgrimages to see him. But he remained, in the words of his biographer, 'a confirmed white racist as well as an unrepentant anti-Semite and pro-fascist'.[57] His last public appearance was at the Savage Club in 1965, where he delivered a speech at the Annual Literature evening. The topic was censorship and he spoke about his role in publishing a clandestine edition of Lawrence's *Lady Chatterley's Lover* during his time in London. After the speech, Stephensen rose to acknowledge the standing ovation from his audience and fell down dead in his chair.[58]

———

One day back in 1941 the journalist Bartlett Adamson had bumped into Stephensen in the street and had asked him what excuse he had for still being alive. Stephensen was outraged and claimed that the contribution he and William had made to Australia was one of martyrdom: 'a sacrifice someone in Sydney had to make to break the spell of democratic decadence which was reducing Sydney's cultural life . . . to a dead level of colonial-provincial inertia.' Rather than being reviled as traitors, the nation should 'cherish the presence of an intransigent in a retrogressing community'.[59] It was the same image Stephensen had used to describe Bee in the foreword he had written for her in 1937 and echoed the claims she sometimes made in defence of her own subversive behaviour.

But Stephensen was not cherished and the charge of disloyalty that remained with him throughout his internment and in the findings of the Clyne Inquiry must have seemed a bitter irony for one who had written and spoken so much about loyalty to Australia first. What neither he nor William ever fully grasped was the way that loyalty was so profoundly binary in the first half of the twentieth century. Most Australians felt proud of their country as part of the British Empire, not distinct from it. In the pre- and post-war periods, Australians were British citizens who travelled overseas on British passports, and this remained the case until 1949.[60] For most citizens, the reassuring flipside of loyalty to Britain was racial homogeneity and the maintenance of a vulnerable white population, so geographically distant from its 'mother country'. This was a further irony for the architects of Australia First who had positioned race and place—the 'genius loci'—in the centre of their rhetoric. Paramilitary organisations like the Old Guard evaded pubic and judicial examination because, despite their volatility, they retained an allegiance to the established order and to Empire above everything else; in doing so, they enjoyed clandestine government support.[61]

Both Stephensen and William consistently denied that they were fascists, claiming they were Australian nationalists. Without doubt they were oppositionists, believing that it was the function and duty of special individuals to influence the broader community as public intellectuals. Bee had expressed similar views about the role of the critic. But it was also an idea shared and reshaped by intellectuals across the broader spectrum of fascist ideology. For Stephenson, more so than for William, the struggle to find a balance between the pre-ordained rights of the artist tyrant and the dynamic will of nationhood—that by its very definition subsumed the individual—was never reconciled. They both maintained what was essentially an elitist view of the artist not only as an arbiter of national culture but also as a political dissenter. In his attempt to merge aesthetics with action Stephensen was following a pattern laid down by the Italian Futurists, path-makers of European fascism. The fact that he used an imported model to develop what was basically a xenophobic and isolationist essay was again an indication of his—and William's—contradictory personalities. Writing to his old publishing partner and now-Marxist writer Jack Lindsay, 26 years after he drafted the essay that began his journey to the Far Right, he referred to Croce, who had supported but then rejected the cultural foundations of fascism:

> In literature as in politics I am for genius loci and for the individual ... if I must be classified I am a Nietzschean Bakuninite! Better say simply an Individualist ... unregimental. In literary evaluations, I stand on Croce's Aesthetic: the creative artist is alone, cannot belong, must swim against the stream.[62]

We can only speculate as to what might have happened to Stephensen had he not come under the yoke of William Miles' political ambitions. Stephensen was always interested in politics but his first enduring commitment was to Australian literature. Initially he had thought that access to William's considerable financial resources might provide another avenue to continue his own publishing ambitions, but over time these became submerged by William's single-minded political pursuits. In both personality and psychological make-up they were very different, and there is no sense of a friendship or even an affection between them, as there was between Stephensen and Jack Lindsay. They both served each other's needs, but it was clear that William, even in his dying days, was in control of the relationship.

For Bee, a witness to her father's failed quest and Stephensen's public humiliation, the attraction of their nationalism would remain but would be qualified by her own isolation. She eventually came to see Stephensen as a traitor who brought her father's reputation into public disrepute, but she had more in common with him than she cared to admit. Like Stephensen, she saw a special role for certain individuals—her aristocracy of genius—in shaping public opinion. Like him, she was attracted to aesthetics on one hand and anarchy and dissent on the other. Like him, she had been locked away for three years. Like him she was financially dependent on William. And like him, there was a quixotic quality to her quest for absolute freedom. But for Bee, watching it all unfold from the margins, there were different windmills to tilt.

12

A Tenant of the City

'Sydney is the best city in Australia to live in and of that city
I prefer the lovely district . . . Kings Cross especially when
the trees are bursting with green exuberance, where priggery
is permanently at the lowest tide.'

Bee Miles 'I Go on a Wild Goose Chase', p. 53

On a crisp autumn evening in March 1945, Bee lay on the porch
of St James' Church waiting for sleep, or the police, whichever
would come first. Gathered around her were her meagre possessions—her blankets, her sandwich board advertising Shakespeare
recitations and her leather schoolbag, containing her manuscripts
and her treasured copies of Swift and Mencken and Shakespeare's
work—she had been reciting set pieces since childhood.

Covered only by a blanket and an old great coat, she lay there on
the hard stone porch while the city sighed and murmured around
her. Diagonally opposite was St Mary's Cathedral, where her father
had sung in the choir as a young man and her grandmother, once
the finest contralto in the colony, had honed her skills in an earlier
time. The view opposite, to the Hyde Park Barracks, was not so different from what her great-grandparents would have seen standing in
the same spot after their marriage in this very church newly built,

a hundred years before. The dynasty they founded had created wealth and prestige. It had built fine houses and flourishing businesses. But all this she had left behind to sleep on the cold hard steps of St James'.

Was it choice or circumstances that had brought Bee here? Possibly it was a combination of the two. The city's wartime accommodation crisis was at its peak, with landlords demanding high prices for rent and 'key money' often beyond the means of average wage earners. But there was also her infamy. Almost every week there was a newspaper report about her and her run-ins with the authorities. No one was going to rent a room to Bee Miles.

And so Bee turned to the city itself for shelter—the city she loved above all others. Its public heart became her home, its streets and steps her bed. She called herself a tenant of the city and for the next twenty years she would remain in its embrace—despite the best efforts of the city fathers and the police to extricate her.

Inevitably the police did come that night, as she knew they would. Despite her protests, they bundled her into a police car and took her to a cell. Later in court, the magistrate ignored Reverend Davidson's evidence that he had granted Bee permission to sleep at the church and the usual charge of offensive behaviour was proved. Bee undertook to stay away from St James'.[1]

———

One of the most common myths about Bee, apart from having a nervous breakdown through over-studying, was that she chose to be homeless. No one chooses to be homeless. Housing shortages in Sydney in the mid-1940s to the 1950s were acute, fuelled by a dearth of building materials, the return of soldiers from the war and an influx of immigrants. In addition, there were large-scale clearances of inner-city areas that had been Bee's domain since the 1920s. Tenants who were lucky enough to be rehoused were placed either in high-rise, low-cost housing or in isolated peri-urban locations with limited transport. For others, particularly older people, homelessness was the only alternative. In 1946 the old age pension was 32 shillings and sixpence, only slightly less than Bee's allowance.[2] Four years later, a Victorian government inquiry found that 15,000 old age pensioners, the majority of whom were women, were living in destitution. Only 2 per cent lived in nursing homes or private institutions.[3] Bee's housing problem had become so acute during the war that, prior to her taking up residence on the porch outside St James', she had installed herself in nearby Sydney Hospital. Insisting she had nowhere else to live, she had spent three weeks moving from ward to ward, chatting and playing cards with the patients. At night she shut herself inside one of the cubicles in the casualty ward. The hospital management, having tried unsuccessfully to remove her, finally resorted to going to court to have her evicted. 'I've nowhere else to live,' she told the magistrate. 'If there's anywhere else, I'll go like a shot.'[4] But there was nowhere. The fact that she had an allowance, as meagre as it was by the 1940s, meant that the city's social services could not help her.

By 1954 the inner-city population had decreased from 400,323 to 365,612.[5] People who could afford it were moving out of the city to the suburbs, which were seen as a healthier alternative. In the years following the Depression and the war, suburban home ownership and domesticity offered stability and security, a notion emphasised increasingly by both Labor and the Liberals. In Menzies' famous 'Forgotten Australians' speech, the home became a metaphor for responsible citizenship. It was the domestic realm, Menzies insisted, the nuclear family and its assets, that modified and directed civic virtues.[6]

While Bee would have agreed with Menzies' focus on self-reliance, she had very different ideas about responsible citizenship. For her it meant living according to the natural laws of simplicity and moral virtue. In Bee's experience, the family home, rather than being a place of nurture and solace, was fraught with danger and violence, from which she sought the safety of public space. 'If anything drove me to my present life,' she remarked, 'it was the fact that I discovered away from home the only formula for happiness.'[7] She also remained faithful to an aesthetic tradition that eschewed the suburbs for the cosmopolitan life of the city. It was the same bohemian aesthetic that decreed that how one lived one's life was an art form. In this way she was able to incorporate the reality of her homelessness into her belief system and not just survive it but make it part of her identity. 'Feather beds,' she wrote, 'are for cops, public servants and other sissies. Clothes and lodging cost me nothing. I sleep under the stars or under the stairs depending on what the weather's like.'[8] Her presence and her physical appearance became visible statements of her aesthetic and, from the 1940s onwards, Bee was linked to the city's public space like no other citizen before or after.

————

The nature of business in post-war Sydney was changing. The decentralisation of industry through the zoning policies of the 1947 Cumberland County Plan, and the rise of motor vehicle ownership, meant a shift in workforce patterns. Not all women returned to purely domestic roles after the war and the growth of clerical and mercantile workers, who were predominantly female, meant an increase in the number of women in the streets of Sydney as both workers and consumers. Although they still faced restrictions in working conditions, unaccompanied women became a more frequent sight and were no longer linked so overtly to prostitution or vagrancy, as they had been before the war. Bee, on the other hand, had been a consistent part of the city's visual landscape for twenty years. In her youth she was the quintessential, if slightly surreal flapper—pushing the boundaries of acceptable female attire with her brief outfits that displayed her bare limbs, exuding sexuality and vigour and revelling in the way her presence unsettled those around her.

Now Bee was in her forties, her appearance had changed dramatically, possibly as an after-effect of the encephalitis lethargica and years of rough living. Photos over a six-year period reveal how much her physical appearance had altered. There is a grainy photograph of Bee taken in 1938 during a parade for the 150th anniversary of the landing of the First Fleet. She is perched on the bonnet of a car smoking a cigarette. In the photo she sits nonchalantly, wearing a brief white tunic, her long tanned legs stretched out in front of her. The caption reads: 'Bea Miles, 36 years old and still slim.' In the mid-1940s the camera caught a very different Bee. She was vast, having gained an enormous amount of weight. Her dress style had changed as well. Images of Bee in the post-war period typically reveal a combination of dresses, men's coats and shoes or bare feet. In a nod to traditional female attire, she occasionally wore a headscarf under her trademark tennis visor. Although she often remarked that she 'liked pretty dresses too', they were beyond her financially and were entirely impractical for the way of life she had adopted.

This was a stark contrast to the way most people dressed in the city. Going to town was an occasion and both men and women dressed formally. Women wore gloves, two-piece suits or frocks with matching handbags and shoes. Everyone wore hats. Newspaper reporters, mostly men, had always been fascinated by Bee's appearance and had once written enthusiastically about her feminine charms. Now the tone had changed. She had become 'mannish', according to journalists. 'Over a spotted skirt she wore a grubby man's sports coat and over that an equally crumpled man's great-coat. On her feet were faded blue slippers. The second little toe of her left foot peaked through a hole in one slipper. This, it can be safely assumed, was not intended to be one of the little touches than enhance the dressing of the chic, well-dressed woman.'[9] Bee herself was more sanguine about the changes to her physical appearance:

> It is very becoming to me to be fat now that I have reached
> a certain age. It is nature's way of telling me to go more
> slowly than I have been accustomed to go and not to

compete with my juniors, not to show jealousy of them and try to steal their thunder. It is no longer my right to receive admiration for a pretty figure. I have had my day. I'm fair fat and nearly fifty. Those men and women over 55 and 35 who are trying to keep their figures slender are suffering from the worst symptom of a filthy disease. The disease is degeneracy not in accordance with nature. The symptom is avoidance of facts. They are avoiding the fact that they are getting old.[10]

Still, Bee was not oblivious to the fact that her appearance created a very different kind of spectacle: 'The worst people I ever met have been the common-place, ulcer-ridden, constipated snobs who travel to town from the stuffy suburbs and shy away from me because I wear an eyeshade, man's coat and carry my swag down Martin Place.'[11] Some of these 'constipated snobs' were her former play-mates who had renounced their bohemian allegiances, like Alma Hood, who decades later recalled her disgust at sighting Bee in the 1950s: 'My last glance of Bea [sic] was when I sat next to her on a bus . . . She was then ugly, fat, dirty and wore a soiled army great-coat and an eye shield . . . Where was the old Bea Miles, I pondered, the girl full of energy and vim in the white frock? There was no trace of her left to the naked eye.'[12]

Despite or even because of the shock value her presence caused, Bee used it to her advantage. Journalists might laugh at her and treat her as an entertainment piece and people might snub her, but along with her notoriety came a certain status. She had become a fixture in the city and that must have given her some sense of security when everything else in her world had changed. Her father was dead. For good or for bad, he had been the centre of her life. The standards he set continued to influence her own philosophical and moral outlook. Stephensen had supported her ambitions as a writer and then betrayed her and was now in exile. Most of her old friends avoided her, finding her an embarrassment. Her financial situation was bleak. The fines she had to pay for both trivial and more serious infringements far exceeded her weekly income. Her brothers, from whom she was estranged, were now in charge of her income and were less likely to top up her finances when she was broke, as her father had done, despite the difficulties in their relationship. And now she was homeless. But Bee was also resilient and, rather than sinking into a hopeless depression, she took stock of her circumstances and began to use her notoriety to her advantage. She returned again to the role she had coveted for so many years, as a public critic, someone to 'set the standards' by which people should live. Ignoring the media's often patronising attitude and knowing that she was considered a good source for material, she used the newspapers to promulgate her message.

In 1948 Bee gave an interview from her temporary accommodation in Rushcutters Bay by the side of a stormwater canal. Sitting snugly in her cave like a modern-day Diogenes,[13] she told the reporter from the *Daily Telegraph* that the 'highest good to which man can obtain is happiness through simplicity and virtue'. She had discovered this truth at the age of 29. What she didn't tell the reporter was that it was also the time she had finally escaped from Parramatta Mental Hospital and her father's control and was living happily in Bohemia. Instead, in a wide-ranging interview, she spoke about the changes she would make if she were dictator of Australia instead of Prime Minister Chifley. These included silencing anyone who placed a stigma on illegitimate children and giving 'big prizes' to the largest and healthiest Australian families. In her own idiosyncratic way, she was reflecting the government's post-war 'populate or perish' mantra. She also discussed questions around her own sanity. 'I am what the average man calls mad—and that admission proves one thing. I cannot be insane at all because no insane person will admit insanity . . . the truth is that he (the average man) just cannot understand me.' Whether the reporter understood her or not is unclear, but he did include her latest manifesto with the article, her 'Rules for Living':

1 Avoid covetousness, envy, greed, jealousy, lying, malice and vindictiveness

2 Be content with what you've got financially, socially and materially

3 Make such provision that you are not forced to live in abject poverty

4 If you are a woman, cry when you are unhappy or in pain—but a man must never cry

5 Drink only when you are thirsty and then only milk, water or soda

6 Eat only when you are hungry

7 Laugh only to show a feeling of pleasure and amusement—but not pleasure or amusement at the predicaments of others

8 Sing when you're happy

9 Sleep when it's dark

10 Don't give a rap for appearances, clothes, money, social position, or what people think of your manners, fashions or traditions

11 Cut your possessions to a minimum

12 If you are a woman, give way to your harmless, rational, material impulses and emotions—but a man must restrain all these

13 Vary your life as much as possible

14 Live toughly, dangerously, excitingly, exhilaratingly and simply

15 Remember the past and try to profit by its lessons; live in the present and try to prepare for the future.[14]

The interview was syndicated and appeared in newspapers across the country. The next morning people in Boyup Brook, Western Australia were reading Bee's advice on how to improve their lives over their tea and toast.

———

'Sydney Diary' was a weekly newspaper column written by the novelist and journalist George Johnston. One week he devoted a ten-minute observation to Bee as she moved through busy city traffic. Describing her as 'that fabulous identity', he observed Bee 'strolling down the middle of George Street . . . reading a highbrow magazine':

> She smiled nicely at the traffic cop, who said 'Hy-ya Bee'. Bee strolled on. It wasn't until an approaching tram came to a shuddering standstill a few inches in front of her that Bee looked up from the article. She smiled at the driver and clambered on to the footboard just beside his compartment—her favourite spot. At Hunter Street a second traffic cop saw her climb from the tram and stand in the middle of George Street while she thumbed through the magazine in search of another article. He told her to get off the road and stop holding the traffic up. She looked at him disdainfully, clambered aboard another tram. She perched nonchalantly on the footboard and looked right through the policeman. A third cop knew the drill. He approached her courteously, said he hoped 'the good lady will make herself comfortable in a seat inside the tram'. Bee flashed him a radiant smile, climbed inside, sat down and opened her magazine. The tram rattled off. And the funny thing is that hundreds of workers who'd missed their trains to watch Bee for ten minutes all went home happy as Larry.[15]

By the 1940s Bee's fame had reached celebrity status. It is difficult to convey just how well known she had become. She was in the news constantly, where even what she shopped for was reported. On one occasion 'Column 8' in the *Sydney Morning Herald* went with a single sentence 'saw Bea on a tram do the *Herald* crossword in two minutes flat'.[16] For the reading public she no longer required context or introduction. When she was absent from the city for more than a week, articles speculated on where she might be; in the last years of the war a newspaper poll had announced Bee was better known than the prime minister. Writing in the *Sydney Morning Herald*, Gavin Souter claimed that 'Miss Miles is surely Sydney's most famous citizen . . . Bea has been seen and heard in the flesh . . . by more people than anyone else in Sydney'.[17] She was constantly being observed—on trams, on buses, in the street. People were always watching Bee, and the fascination followed her wherever she went. Syndicated articles had made her famous across the country, so when she travelled outside Sydney, her visits attracted media attention. In 1944 she spent several months in Mildura. When she left the town in December, her departure was covered by the *Barrier Daily Truth*, which described her final bus journey through the town as if she were a departing celebrity. Wellwishers had given her money, cigarettes, biscuits and chocolates for the journey, she told the paper, for which she was very grateful. She thanked the town for its hospitality.[18]

As Johnston's article indicates, there was a large element of performance in the way Bee moved around the city, and although she continually claimed to despise all actors, and that she never wanted to be 'known', she also admitted that 'everyone likes an audience'.[19] After all performance and theatricality were in her blood. She'd had a close relationship with her grandmother Ellen, a renowned concert performer who had spent her professional life surrounded by theatrical people. Her father had sung regularly in choirs and had given public performances from Shakespeare's plays. He had also performed as a political speaker and travelled the country on speaking tours when she was growing up. In a way it was a logical step for her to utilise her natural talent and her vast knowledge of Shakespeare to try to supplement her income through performance.

It's difficult to pinpoint exactly when Bee began offering poetry and drama recitations for money, but her sandwich board advertising Shakespeare, prose and poetry recitals at various prices ranging from sixpence to three shillings became a familiar sight from post-war period onwards. Her repertoire also included Swift, Mencken, Nietzsche and Kipling, though these were rarer as she disliked reciting non-Australian prose. She would move around the city during the day, to various select spots and set up her board. The steps of the Mitchell Library, opposite the Botanic Gardens and the Shakespeare monument her father had helped to raise money for, were an ideal spot as she could be sure of a regular flow of students coming in and out of the library. Unlike her father or his socialist colleagues, she didn't require a soapbox at the Domain to attract an interested crowd. Wherever she was, outside the State Theatre or on the library steps, Bee drew people and held her audiences spellbound. On a good day she could earn up to seven shillings.

In 1947 Bee took her performance to another level when she entered the Sydney Eisteddfod. The Eisteddfod, which continues today, began in 1933 and was a showcase for aspiring actors, singers, poets, writers and musicians, who performed in competitive heats at venues around the city, including the Town Hall. During the post-war period, events were well attended and winners were awarded cash prizes. Bee entered the Scene from Shakespeare event, choosing a scene from *Measure for Measure*, the same play her parents had performed for the Shakespeare Society in 1912. The scene she selected required three parts and she performed all of them herself in full costume. She earned 79 marks out of 100, with the adjudicator noting that she was 'a first-class comedy actress'. Although formally disqualified, she received an honourable mention.[20] The next year the papers announced that she was the first person to enter the verse-speaking championship and would recite the 'The Swallow' by Wilfred Gibson. But when the Eisteddfod came round, she refused to recite the set piece, preferring to use two poems by the Australian poet Ian Mudie—a former protégée of her father and Stephensen. She wrote to the adjudicator beforehand, explaining that other than Shakespeare, she would not recite English poetry to an Australian audience. On the day of the contest, she was arrested for poking her tongue out at a lorry driver who refused to give her a lift. She told journalists outside the court that she had been given permission to perform that evening, even though she would be disqualified for not reciting Gibson's poem. She was praised for her performance and given another certificate of merit. The court fined her five shillings.[21]

———

Bee had always loved the theatre and had been attending opera and symphony concerts since she was a child. She was fascinated by the physicality of conductors on stage. The few surviving pieces of music criticism she wrote describe in intricate detail the various gestures conductors used to coax the music from their orchestras. She was a common sight during opera and symphony seasons, where she liked to sit as closely as possible to the conductor. This was not always welcomed by the artist.

On one occasion, when the world-famous pianist Claudio Arrau was preparing for a concert at the Town Hall, Bee sat on the floor listening to his warm-up, while playing a game of patience. She was removed by a policeman but returned later during the concert and sat on the stage. When approached by the police, she scrambled over some rows and tried to wrestle a man for his seat. She was arrested and fined £5. It would have been cheaper for her to buy a seat in the stalls.[22]

Other outings were more successful. During a Let's Make Opera production, patrons, both adults and children, were grouped into different sections as part of the chorus. Some were to be owls, others herons or turtle-doves. Just before the concert commenced, Bee complained that she preferred the role of the turtle-dove to that of an owl. The conductor acquiesced and the whole audience waited while Bee made her way slowly up from the stalls to the mezzanine seats. The performance was a success and afterwards she sent a huge box of chocolates backstage for the child performers.

Although Bee preferred silent movies and, above all, Chaplin's *Modern Times* to 'talkies', she was an avid cinema-goer during the 1940s and 1950s. She attended all first releases in cinemas throughout the city and Kings Cross and was given admission without charge. There were times when she strained the goodwill of cinema proprietors, particularly when she smoked. Another problem arose when Bee disliked the film and inflicted her views loudly on the other patrons. She became particularly incensed when actors kissed with their mouths open. Curiously, there is no record of how she responded to the requirement for audiences to stand during the national anthem, which was still 'God Save the Queen'. On several occasions Bee was brought to court on charges of offensive behaviour, but these were generally dismissed when she claimed that she was merely offering her critical view, which was technically correct. Once she became violent when she had bought a ticket but was refused entry to a new release at the St James Theatre. It was claimed that she hit one usher in the stomach and stomped on the foot of another. In court the manager acknowledged that she had enjoyed free entry for at least seven years. She was fined a hefty £22 for assault, smoking and indecent language.[23]

Far more humiliating than being evicted from the cinema or the theatre was the charge of begging that Bee received during a Sydney Symphony concert in the Domain in 1950. She was spotted by police approaching several groups of people and asking them 'to spare a penny'. When asked by the police why she was begging she responded, 'What a stupid question, you stupid nincompoop.' She told the court that she was not begging but collecting donations for the orchestra. 'It was a very mild way of showing our appreciation.' She had collected eight pence and added sixpence of her own. She had been unable to give the collection to the orchestra straight away because she had been arrested and held in the cells. She had paid it after she was released on bail and had brought the receipt to court for evidence. Despite Bee's explanations and the receipt, the magistrate found the charge proved—but he discharged her immediately afterwards. Journalists recorded her obvious indignation, pointing out that although she had been arrested over 100 times by that stage, she had never faced a begging charge before.[24]

———

Standing in the dock one day, Bee was asked to state her occupation. Along with the usual response of 'student', she added 'peripatetic' and 'old and fat'. 'Peripatetics,' she told the Appeals Court, 'were the original Greek philosophers who moved about in circles. I am like my father; he was a peripatecian [sic] also.'[25] Although Bee was often spotted in the outer suburbs of Sydney, there was a certain circularity to her movements when she was in the centre of town. She would wake at five and hook her blankets to her belt—the cestus she had used on her epic trips in the 1930s. She would leave whatever location she had been sleeping in at the time, the cave at Rushcutters Bay or the ground under a shed in the Domain, and make her way across to the Mason's Café in Elizabeth Street, opposite Central Station. She ate breakfast there every day for nearly twenty years and always had the same meal—steak and eggs.[26]

After breakfast Bee would walk down a few blocks to the corner of Reservoir and Elizabeth Streets, to Dobson's Turkish Bathhouse. Turkish bathhouses were a feature of Victorian Sydney that remained popular until the mid-twentieth century, particularly for working people living in rooms or boarding houses around the city. Women could bathe in a separate area or at a designated time of day. There was a common perception during the 1940s and 1950s, when Bee was sleeping rough, that she was unclean and therefore possibly diseased. In fact, courtesy of the bathhouse owner, Mr Dobson, Bee had her own designated timeslot—between 7.00 and 7.30 every morning, where she bathed and dressed and dried her hair.[27] Both her father and Hesling had commented on her obsession with bathing and her preference for long, hot baths. Despite her current state of homelessness, she had managed to continue the practice.

After her bath Bee would don her sandwich board, advertising her services as a recitalist, and head down to Eddy Avenue near Belmore Park. On the way she would call at a delicatessen for a free bottle of milk and be given a free piece of fruit from a fruit barrow. If there was a mounted policeman on duty, she would always stop to nuzzle his horse and feed it a carrot or some sugar. The mounted police was one of the few sections of the police force with whom Bee had a cordial relationship.[28] From Eddy Avenue she might take a bus out to Watsons Bay, at the ocean's edge. She wasn't taking the bus ride for the scenery or to pass the time—this was work. She would sometimes approach passengers to see if they wanted to hear a recital, but more often she would ask them if they were interested in a wager. If they said yes, she would bet with them on how many taxis they might see between the next bus top and Watsons Bay. She was usually right, and the passenger paid up. Bus conductors tended to turn a blind eye.[29]

Arriving back in the city, Bee would make her way to the steps of the Mitchell Library where she would continue to ply her trade. She had been banned from the reading rooms for smoking, but the librarians tolerated her presence on the front steps. She would often stand at Bebarfald's Corner, opposite the Town Hall, though this was less fruitful due to the constant presence of the police.[30] Towards the end of the afternoon, she might visit a few select acquaintances, including an ambulance driver at Sydney Hospital. She borrowed books from the Municipal Library and occasionally visited the bookshops in Elizabeth Street. Her reading material, like her movements, was circular: Shakespeare, Swift, Voltaire, Xavier Herbert and Norman Douglas. She was particularly fond of Swift and had memorised all three languages from *Gulliver's Travels*, which she could still speak in her seventies.[31] Beyond that select group of writers, she was not interested in fiction. The texts she considered indispensable were Mencken's *Chrestomathy* and dictionaries—biographical, etymological and historical. A well-educated person needed to read only ten books, she contended.[32]

Depending on what was playing at the time, Bee would go to the cinema. She disliked comedies and preferred westerns like *High Noon* or dramas like *The Big Heat*. Occasionally she might visit a newspaper office and provide them with an interview or a press release on her subject of choice, which varied from euthanasia rights to sexual freedom, the fallibility of the justice system or the uselessness of the monarchy. At 5 p.m. she would have her dinner: curried tongue and peas. She'd been eating the same dinner every evening for many years and was not inclined to vary her diet. Her allowance, which was still controlled by her brothers, was around £3 and 10 shillings (or 70 shillings) a week. She could live on fifteen shillings a day but could reduce it to seven shillings if things were tight, as they often were. This included food, newspapers, cigarettes—she smoked two packets a day—shoe repairs every now and then and a haircut every three months.[33] She wore the same clothes until they wore out and shopped at thrift shops when she needed new ones. Bee was living below the poverty line, and the money she earned from reciting and gambling was vital to being able to maintain even this fairly spartan existence. Her perambulations now complete, she would retire to her chosen spot for the night at 6 p.m. It was a simple routine with little variation, as she traced and retraced her steps over the public heart of the city, engraving her presence onto the memories of its citizens.

———

Bee had several regular spots in the city that she would use to sleep, along with the Rushcutters Bay cave and the Domain shed. In the winter of 1952, the new headmaster at Darlinghurst School discovered that Bee, through an arrangement with the cleaner, had been sleeping in a timber demountable. The cleaner had even lit the fire for her. The headmaster, Donald McLean, who later went on to become the *Sydney Morning Herald*'s education correspondent, knew Bee by sight and reputation, but hadn't realised she was also a resident at his school. Surprisingly, he tolerated her presence until, later in the summer, she moved under the girls' classroom and a teacher complained. When he approached her, he found her snugly tucked up under the stairs. Informing her that he had received complaints about her, she responded:

> If I am traduced by ignorant tongues
> which neither know
> My faculties or my person, yet will be
> The chronicle of my doing, let me say
> 'Tis but the fate of place and the rough brake
> That virtue must go through.[34]

This rather startled the headmaster, who then decided to use bribery rather than logic. He offered her two shillings, and as she took the money she declared, 'My poverty not my will consents.' Recognising this quote from *Romeo and Juliet*, he was able to respond: 'I pay thy poverty and not thy will.' Now it was Bee's turn to be surprised. 'Good Lord,' she declared. 'Tongues in the trees, books in the running brooks, sermons in stones and good old Will in a schoolmaster.' As the headmaster was escorting her off the premises, they passed a group of students painting a mural of the world map on the schoolyard wall. Bee was silent for a moment and then proclaimed:

> How many goodly creatures are
> There here!
> How beauteous mankind is. O
> Brave new world
> That has such people in it.[35]

This was a far more gracious eviction than her usual encounters. Believing that it was safer to sleep outside than in buildings, particularly empty ones, Bee sometimes used bandstands in city parks. In fact, she only recorded one incident where she came close to being sexually assaulted. She confronted her would-be attacker by asking, 'You're not going to molest old Bee Miles are you?' 'Are you Bee Miles?' the man responded, and then shook her hand.[36] But it wasn't the public who posed a threat to her safety: it was the police. When Bee was sleeping in the cave at Rushcutters Bay, the police didn't tend to harass her with any consistency—possibly because she was out of public view. But when she relocated to the more conspicuous location of Belmore Park, her presence was far more visible. She was sleeping in the bandstand in the middle of the park and, as the police conducted their nightly rounds, they would often target her, jumping on her, kicking off her blankets, throwing her shoes away and, if she was sleeping on a bench, tipping her onto the ground. Occasionally, and most degradingly, they would urinate on her.[37] Finally, it became too much, and Bee sought sanctuary at nearby Christ Church St Laurence.

Walking down George Street from Central Station, it is easy to pass Christ Church St Laurence without even noticing it. Designed by the colonial architect Edmund Blacket and consecrated in 1845, it is the one of the oldest churches in Sydney, its weathered spire still peeking out over a crowded city-scape. Once dominating the surrounding paddocks and church school, its land has been gradually subsumed by the ever-encroaching city. Now only the church and rectory remain, sitting like a strange island enclosed on all sides by buildings, traffic and noise. Over the years this church has served the city's wealthy and its poor and been the source of both controversy and opposition. Perhaps the most controversial period was between the 1930s and the 1960s, under the leadership of Father John Hope.

Hope, a descendent of Samuel Marsden and uncle to Manning Clark, was an Anglo Catholic in an era when the divide between Catholics and Protestants was rigidly maintained. Conservative Anglican bishops were highly suspicious of this priest who embraced not only the rituals of the 'scarlet woman of Rome' but was also an overt adopter of Christian socialism. Amongst his parishioners were a young Margaret Throsby, Patrick White, the author Kylie

Tennant and her husband Lewis Rodd. Rodd, who wrote a bio-graphy of Father Hope, described him as 'young, handsome, gay and reckless . . . during his 38 years at the parish he was subject to a campaign of ecclesiastical bigotry and persecution never directed against any other priest of the Church of England in Australia'.[38] Along with Bee, he was a well-known figure in Sydney and had more than a penchant for controversy.

One Sunday morning after mass, Father Hope headed for the clergy house for breakfast. With him was a young man called John Pollard, who boarded at the clergy house and performed church duties during services. As they entered the porch, they almost stepped on a body lying there covered in a tarpaulin, with a mop of hair protruding from one end. Father Hope, who'd assumed it was a homeless man, was surprised when a cultured female voice emerged from the coverings, 'I know who you are, you're Father John. What's for breakfast?'[39] It was the beginning of a relationship that would continue for a decade.

Over the years Father Hope was often called out in the middle of the night to defend Bee against police charges or pay a fine so she wouldn't have to go to gaol.[40] In the beginning she slept on the porch between the clergy house and the vestry, so that the priests would have to step over her. She was comfortable there, having long preferred to sleep on the ground rather than a bed. Occasionally she would join in the conversations emanating from the clergy house, if the subject was of interest, or she might provide a lecture of her own on rationalism. At other times, she would come through the side door of the church, where she would sit on what was known as the drunks' pew, often still wearing her sandwich board, and smoking a cigarette.

Sometimes Bee might wander up the southern aisle on her way to the vestry and sit in the front pew to listen to the sermon, the sound of her unlaced sandshoes slapping the floor tiles as she walked, her great coat swishing around her.[41] If it looked like she was going to interject, a church warden would entice her outside for a discussion. But she didn't interject. She knew the structure of the mass and respected its solemnity. After mass it would be a different story. Assuming the rationalist mantle, she would engage in debate with church regulars as well as visiting dignitaries with equal gusto. There was a theatricality about her speeches, John Pollard remembered. She loved to be the centre of attention and the more attention she received the more outrageous her statements became.[42] She would often stand just outside the church and affirm her atheism—just in case anyone had forgotten. On one occasion Pollard remembered her loudly declaring 'Homosexuality is not dirty', clearly and deliberately sounding out each word. In an era of homosexual panic, when gay men and women risked arrest, imprisonment and irreparable damage to their lives, it would have been a reassuring statement.[43] (But it would also be contradicted in some of her later writing, where she used the trope of homosexuality to question Australian masculinity.)

On Sunday evenings the church held youth meetings. John Lee, who was then a young student, was a regular attendant. For him Bee was a rather frightening figure. 'Who are you?' she would boom, along with other questions, which he felt impelled to answer in case she became angry, although she never did. Occasionally the priest conducting the youth group meetings would call Bee in and ask her to perform some Shakespeare. The group was 'awestruck'.[44] Father Jim Brady, who ran the group, remembered that Bee would often stay around for tea 'taking up more than half the couch, throwing cigarette butts all over the room and delivering discourses on her favourite themes'.[45]

Once a year Christ Church St Laurence would conduct a Dedication Festival Procession to commemorate the church's consecration. It was a tradition reaching back to its earliest days. The entire congregation, clergy and church attendants would walk around the parish boundaries—now much reduced—stopping at different locations to say a prayer. In the past the procession had been accompanied by a brass band; even in the 1950s, it was still a spectacular event.[46]

Bee, who claimed to dislike processions, but always seemed to be in the middle of them, was photographed once, marching with the faithful and trying to shield her identity with a piece of paper.

It was a fascinating relationship—the avowed and proud atheist and the devout priest, intransigent and defiant in his faith. Lewis Rodd described Bee as Father Hope's hairshirt, but there was a kind of reciprocity in their relationship. They admired and respected each other's principles and intellect, echoing the collaboration between her father and Daniel Mannix during the anti-conscription campaigns. They both understood that life's trajectory was not a straight line, but a multitude of possible side streets and alleyways, where its true richness and meaning could be found. And there was genuine affection between them. Often a serious man, whenever Bee's name was mentioned, Father Hope would throw his head back and laugh.[47] When he was recovering in hospital after a serious illness, the first visitors allowed to see him were the archbishop—and Bee. But Father Hope also worried about his famous tenant. Her kidneys were not in good shape and the cold marble floor of the porch was contributing to her growing incontinence.

One winter when Bee was facing a particularly serious charge for snapping the hinges off a taxi door, Father Hope decided not to pay her bail. 'She will be all the better off for a thorough clean-up and a stay in Long Bay over the winter,' he said.[48] Bee was away for four-and-a-half months; when she returned it was decided that she would sleep in the laundry. Unfortunately, this was directly under Father Hope's window, and Bee's constant visits to the bathroom often kept him awake through the night. Father Hope gave her a key, which also opened the gate, so she could come and go independently and she had her meals provided, which would be passed through a window of the kitchen. She remained at the church until Father Hope's retirement in 1964.

Throughout the 1940s and 1950s, Bee continued to enjoy a kind of celebrity status in Sydney and beyond. Nationally syndicated articles and reports about her ensured that her profile was maintained for readers across the country. Ironically, despite all their money and resources, her father and Stephensen were never able to achieve the same audience reach as Bee did. Her visible presence in the city was a touchstone for its residents, a reassuring link with the past in an environment that was changing rapidly around them. And with the fame came a certain security. More important than the free entry into cinemas and the occasional free produce was her belief that she was unlikely to be locked up in an asylum again. She was confident that the psychiatrists had finally found her incurable. It was in these post-war years that Bee felt more secure than she had since childhood: 'I could not live in any other city than Sydney. Not only is it the most interesting city, it has the most temperate climate. Besides that I have a great many privileges here; so the police may as well cease trying to put me out.'[49]

The trouble was, they didn't.

13

Transport Wars

'Am I mad because I don't want to sleep in a feather bed?
Am I a psychopath because I don't drink? Am I wonky in
the belfry because I'm not and never have been a prostitute?
Am I loony because I refuse charity? Am I off my head
because I like riding in taxi-cabs?'

Bee Miles, 'The Cops and Me', p. 7

James Homes stepped off the boat in Circular Quay and hailed a
taxi, heading for his destination in Bondi Junction. A first-time
visitor to the harbour city, he didn't realise he had already offended
the taxi driver by sitting in the back seat. As the taxi idled in traffic,
he noticed a large, dishevelled woman sitting on the step of the tram
opposite, holding some newspapers. Then, in matter of seconds, she
was in the taxi with them. For a large woman she could move fast, he
thought. Unlike James, she sat in the front seat. Slightly confused,
he sat back in his seat: perhaps this was the way people caught taxis
in Sydney? But his confusion turned to horror when the taxi driver
took hold of the woman's head and banged it repeatedly against the
passenger door frame. The woman looked at the driver and pushed
her full weight against him, sending him back towards the driver's

206

side of the taxi. 'I'm in now,' she told him. 'Here, have a paper.' Was this a domestic, James wondered, moving even further back in his seat. He'd been told Sydney was a tough town; maybe this *was* how they did things.

With his additional passenger now firmly ensconced in the front seat, the driver took off and headed straight to Martin Place, pulling up beside the GPO. He left the taxi and sprinted over to a policeman, mounted on a white horse. But the woman was quicker. She exited the cab and ran up the steps of the GPO, disappearing into its vast interior. When the driver returned, he appeared calmer. 'That was Bee Miles,' he told his passenger, who was still recovering from the shock. After learning that James was new to Sydney, he proceeded to educate him about his famous passenger. Apparently, he was quite the authority. Bee was, he told him, 'a real character'. She lived in a drain somewhere out by La Perouse. She'd been a real brain but she'd studied too hard at university and went off her rocker. Her father was a judge and paid her to keep away from him. Now she went around spouting Shakespeare for threepence. She always had a crowd around her. As they proceeded through the traffic, the driver wound down his window and shouted, 'Just had Bee Miles in me cab,' to every taxi he passed. He seemed almost jubilant. When they finally reached their destination, he told his passenger, 'Don't forget, mate, you've been in a cab with Bee Miles.'[1]

———

Fame can be a two-headed beast. On one hand the general population had shown a huge affection for Bee. She represented an aspect of Australian culture—a rebellious spirit—that tapped into something deep within the nation's consciousness, despite the ever-increasing thrall of post-war conformity and consumerism. On the other hand, her intransigence, her refusal to 'capitulate', fed her notoriety, and made her a target of an overzealous police force and a public enemy of the transport system. As the 1950s progressed, her confrontations with both these entities would become more intense.

From the beginning of her time as a university student Bee had maintained a fascination with movement and risk. She was in perpetual motion, always travelling from one location to the next, whether it was to another suburb or another state. And she was impatient. Apart from when she was sleeping, the idea of waiting, of staying still, was anathema. But it was more than impatience, it was a compulsion that she recognised, and like her homelessness, incorporated into her aesthetic. Harmless impulses, according to her 'Formula for Happiness', should be given into, in the same way that life should be lived 'toughly, dangerously, excitingly, exhilarat-ingly and simply'. Risk was also part of her father's legacy—he had always been prepared to take enormous risks to pursue his goals.

When she was younger and suppler, Bee had been drawn to the exhilaration that leaping onto cars and trains and moving trams produced. She loved the transgressive nature of her actions and the shock value they created in drivers and spectators. It was all part of 'the game'. Now she was older and, although she could still move quickly, she wasn't able to leap onto moving vehicles as she had in the past. Bee continued to use trams and buses but tended to board them in a more conventional way—though she could swing between moving trams if she needed to, sometimes two or three at a time. Once inside however, and in a confined space, confrontations inevitably erupted.

Trams had been part of the city's fabric since 1861, when the first horse-drawn cars were introduced, running along Pitt Street from Circular Quay to the Railway Terminus at Redfern (which preceded Central Station). These early conveyances were soon replaced by steam-driven motorised trams, imported especially for the 1879 International Exhibition held in the Garden Palace at the Botanic Gardens. Although the new trams were an immediate success and were seen as the apex of modern technology, by 1906 they were replaced by an even newer innovation—the electric tramcar. With a vast network of tracks extending through the city and surrounding suburbs as far as Naremburn in the north and La Perouse at the city's southern-most reach, commuters embraced the 'toast racks', as they were known, as an essential feature of a bustling, modern city. With over 290 kilometres of track—the most in the British Empire—trams conveyed commuters to work during the week and to racecourses, dances, beaches and picnic spots on weekends. In 1939, at the outbreak of war, trams transported 300 million passengers per year across Sydney. By 1945 the number had risen to 400 million. In their heyday trams were Sydney's most popular and reliable means of transport.[2]

The interior design of trams was simple and quite intimate. Each end of the tram had a driver's compartment, which was separated from the rest of the tram by a glass partition. The compartment was raised above the rest of tram, so the driver had to step up to enter his section. The rest of tram comprised of rows of seats that held eight passengers, who sat facing each other in close proximity. Smoking compartments were available at each end of the tram, with pull-up blinds. These were mostly occupied by men. Within the car, sections were separated by sliding glass doors. A footboard ran along the outside of the tram, which the conductors used to move between cars to collect the fares.[3]

Like most people living in Sydney in the interwar period Bee used trams on a daily basis. Newly appointed tram drivers and conductors would be given her description and told not to bother to try to collect her fare. Bee's seat of preference was on the driver's step or the footboard, considered 'no go zones' for the public. At other times she would sit in the smoking carriage, where she had a favourite seat. If it was already occupied by another passenger, she would demand that they vacate 'her' seat, to which they usually acquiesced. The general attitude, one former tram driver recalled, was 'amused tolerance'.[4] The police and magistrates did not always share the same benevolent view. In 1944 Bee told a magistrate that she had been riding around the city for free for seventeen years.

She knew all the conductors and only three refused to allow her free transport. It was the same with the inspectors, the 'kellys'. Only two chose to ignore the tacit agreement between Bee and the tram system. It was part of the broader contract Bee believed she had with the city; large sections of the public and the transport system believed it too. It was only when certain individuals challenged the agreement that things became confrontational.

It started with hats. Bee had once remarked that the surest way to cause a man to lose his sense of equilibrium was to remove his hat. She had done this with a policeman in 1941. He had taken her writing pad—something that would have outraged her—and in retaliation she took his hat and kicked it across busy William Street.[5] It was the beginning of a trend. In December of the same year, just a month before her father died, she had been writing in a tram and claimed not to have seen the conductor, who was demanding her fare. He had reached into her pocket and taken her hairbrush. In retaliation Bee took his cap. The conductor then threw her hairbrush out of the tram window. In response, she threw his cap out after it. The magistrate, while dismissing the charges, declared that she was 'a public nuisance'. Over the next five years two more similar incidents occurred, including one in which Bee walked along the tram's external footboard to the driver's compartment, reached in and removed his cap, knocking his glasses off in the process. What he had done to provoke such a determined response is unrecorded.

While this method of retaliation was reserved for men, Bee's melees with conductresses were far less benign. In 1943 Bee was the only passenger on a late-night tram travelling along William Street to Kings Cross. The conductress, one Lily May Mapstone, was retrieving her coat from the front of the car when she felt a heavy blow from behind. Bee had pushed her because she had ignored her repeated requests to close the sliding compartment door. Lily responded by slapping Bee repeatedly across the face and a violent fight broke out between them. The driver eventually intervened. Later at the tram depot Bee claimed that the driver had held her while someone else 'blackened' her eyes. 'I always try to be proper,' Bee declared to the magistrate, 'but spite always annoys me, especially spite in women. With men it's not so bad.'[6] Five months later there was another violent encounter. The conductress, Elizabeth Kuhn, claimed that Bee had kicked her in the stomach. In court Bee said that she had struck Kuhn after she had called her a 'lunatic' and ordered her to leave the tram, striking her on the forehead. Bee still had the bruise when she was remanded in custody and sent for medical observation. She was later sentenced to three months' gaol. At both hearings it was stated that conductresses across the tram network were afraid of Bee and never asked for her fares.

On the one occasion where Bee was charged with assaulting a passenger, the victim was again female. Dorothy, a science worker from Sydney University, was sitting in a tram at Railway Square on the evening of 26 April 1945. Bee boarded the tram and sat opposite her and immediately asked her fellow passenger to move along so she could put her feet up. When Dorothy refused, Bee raised her feet and allegedly kicked her. During questioning by Bee's solicitor, Dorothy admitted that Bee had been barefoot, and the kick was not hard, and that Dorothy had produced a knife, which she held against Bee's leg. But, after the prosecutor produced a list of Bee's prior convictions, Bee was found guilty of assault and fined £5.[7] This propensity for physical violence seemed to be reserved for women and recalled the violent encounters she experienced during her years in the asylums. Bee had always been proud of her physical strength, and in that oppressive environment she had learnt to use her body as a weapon against violent patients and nurses. It was the same in her forties. If anything, she was stronger now, having become adept at using her increasing bulk as a physical defence or, in some cases, an attack. The papers had begun calling her 'the terror of the trams'.

At the same time there was a curious chivalric thread emerging in Bee's court defences. When questioned about fare evasion she would contend that 'a woman is entitled to get what she can for nothing as long as there are no strings on it: that is an unwritten moral law'.[8] This was a distinct misalignment with her public statements about the importance of independence and self-sufficiency; one newspaper reported it as 'a queer idea', but it did have a basis in the long history of arbitration that enshrined men as breadwinners and women as dependants. Based on the 1908 Harvester decision, which set the minimum wage as adequate for a man with a dependent wife and three children, subsequent rulings reinforced women's dependence on men by prohibiting married women from many areas of the workforce.[9] In areas where women were allowed to work their wages were often set at up to 50 per cent less than their male counterparts. If the state had made Bee a dependant by virtue of her sex, then the state should not expect her to pay for its services. Armed with what she regarded as a rationalist defence, she continued to use the tram system with relative freedom, even sitting in the driver's compartment on occasion, riding on the footboards or swinging between trams when the police were in pursuit.[10] This was a risky practice, though there is only one report of an accident. In 1945 the *Newcastle Morning Herald* reported that Bee had been taken to Sydney Hospital with concussion and internal injuries after she fell from a moving tram as it turned a corner.[11]

Buses presented a different set of challenges. The interior space was far more confined, and Bee couldn't leap from a moving bus like she could from a tram. While most conductors chose not to challenge Bee by trying to collect her fare, there were some notable exceptions. On one occasion an incensed inspector forced an entire busload of passengers to be diverted to Enfield Police Station because Bee refused to pay her fare. The episode cost her £2 in fines. The bus fare would have cost her a few pence.[12] But there was another encounter on a bus that never made its way into the paper—or perhaps journalists found it too indelicate to report.

In 1962 Robert Lidden was a probationary constable assigned to No. 2 Division, Regent Street Police Station. It was his first posting and his first shift. As part of his introduction, his sergeant told him, 'At some stage you will come across a person called Bea Miles. She is mad and usually abuses bus conductors and taxi drivers and refuses to pay her fare. Treat her politely and she will cause you no trouble but try the heavy with her and you'll cop it.' A few months later, Constable Lidden had his first encounter with Bee. It was evening and as he was walking his beat near the bus stop at Railway Square, opposite Central Station, he saw a bus conductor racing towards him calling out, 'It's Bea again, Constable.'

With the conductor in tow, he headed to a stationary green government bus, where two men stood. One was neatly dressed in a suit and tie, with a large ticket inspector's badge on the lapel of his coat. Behind him was the bus driver, with an enormous grin on his face. With a policeman's trained eye, he surveyed the scene.

> The ticket inspector was holding the right leg of his trousers up and I saw that from the shin area down it was wet. I also saw that he was wearing brown shoes and socks and that the right shoe and sock were also very wet. He had a very shocked look on his face ... all he could mutter was 'She ... she ... she ...' I looked at the bus driver who was still grinning and he said, 'It's Bea, mate. He got on here and when he got to Bea she refused to show a ticket, so he got pretty stroppy so she up and pissed on his leg.'

Constable Lidden boarded the bus, where Bee was by now the only passenger. As he walked along the aisle he was greeted by the strong smell of urine and a large wet puddle. 'Good evening, Miss Miles,' he said. 'Good evening, Constable,' she responded. 'Can you tell me what happened?' he asked. 'Well, he abused me because I didn't have a ticket, so I pissed on him. Serves him right,' Bee explained. After agreeing to accompany him, Bee and Constable

Lidden walked to Regent Street Police Station, talking amiably, with the wet-legged ticket inspector following behind. 'Although the incident happened nearly 45 years ago,' Robert recalled:

> the memory of it is still as vivid as if it happened yesterday. The big grin on the bus driver's face, the shocked look of horror on the ticket inspector's face, contemplating his wet trouser leg and shoe . . . My enduring memory of Bea Miles is that of a colourful eccentric person whom if you treated with courtesy she responded in kind. If, however you abused her she could react in a most unexpected manner, as the ticket inspector certainly found out! She certainly had no love or respect for bus conductors, taxi drivers and police, and certainly not officious ticket inspectors![13]

The body, it seems, was still Bee's weapon of choice.

By the 1950s the growth of motor vehicle ownership and successful lobbying by vested interest groups like the National Roads and Motorists' Association (NRMA) saw the demise of trams in pursuit of more 'efficient' transport options. Trams, once seen as an emblem of modernity, were now viewed as anachronistic—perhaps a little like Bee. Modern cities needed freeways, not tram tracks, and, as the overhead electric wires were removed and the tram tracks covered over, the first freeway—the Cahill Expressway—began moving drivers over the bridge and into the city, despite the protests of many of its citizens. But the car was now ubiquitous. Across the country, car registrations had increased from 820,000 in 1939 to 2,500,000 in 1958.[14] The private motor car was king, and Bee was one of its greatest enthusiasts, though not in the way that motoring associations could have ever envisioned.

———

Bee had long ago discovered that the conventional means of hitchhiking—a term she disliked because of its American connotations—didn't really work in Australia. Cars simply didn't stop at the sight of an upraised thumb. It was more effective to approach drivers directly using a technique she called 'hail and ride'. It was a far more elegant phrase, she claimed, and better suited to an Australian setting. She would stand on the edge of the road and attempt to wave cars down. When this proved ineffective, as it often did, she would stand in the middle of the street, forcing cars to swerve around her. It was not without risk, and she was injured several times. In 1947 she was taken to hospital and treated for shock after being hit by a car, and over the next decade the accidents were more frequent.[15] In 1950 she made headlines, when in a nod to modern technology, she bought an autocycle—a type of motorised bicycle—and promptly collided with a car in the centre of the city. She had a learner's permit, probably the only time she'd legally driven anything that had a motor. She was taken to Sydney Hospital and treated for cuts and bruises. The fate of the autocycle is unknown but it quickly disappeared from public view.[16]

Hitchhiking was not illegal in Australia, and by the 1950s it was becoming increasingly common. 'Everywhere you go these days people are hailing cars,' a judge noted as he upheld Bee's appeal against a conviction. The arresting officer in the original charge had told the judge he was 'very offended' when he saw Bee wave her hand over her head to stop a car.[17] Three months prior to Bee's arrest two young men were interviewed by journalists about their hitchhiking adventures around the country, which they said, 'was the easiest thing in the world to do'. They didn't have any trouble getting lifts and free meals and had 'a whale of a time'.[18] Bee's situation was quite different. Even in her time as the much-lauded 'Bumper Bar Beauty' she often had problems getting cars and trucks to stop for her. Now in her forties, with her perceived shabbiness, her large frame and her notoriety, drivers were even more reluctant to stop. And there was also the issue of her gender. Women didn't hitchhike, nor did they wave down cars. She was frequently charged with swearing at drivers, or making rude gestures, including poking out her tongue, when they refused to stop. Other charges included blocking traffic, though she successfully challenged this on appeal, with the judge agreeing that it was not an offence to obstruct traffic if there was a 'reasonable excuse'.[19] It was a short-lived victory. In most cases, Bee was found guilty of offensive behaviour.

Having abandoned her one attempt at conventional transport, and no doubt frustrated by the failure of her 'hail and ride' technique, Bee resorted to an even more direct approach. She would wait until a car was stopped at traffic lights and simply jump into the passenger side, demanding to be taken to her destination. 'Take me to the city,' she would command, in her usual imperious tone. It must have been a startling experience for the drivers; local and interstate papers often published anecdotes by people whose cars had been hijacked by Bee.

On a number of occasions it was startling for Bee as well, when the cars she invaded were driven by off-duty police. On a winter's day in August 1955 Bee jumped into a car on Parramatta Road. Unfortunately for her, the driver was a sheriff's officer, who had a warrant for her arrest. He probably couldn't believe his luck. He drove her straight to Long Bay Prison. She not only had outstanding warrants, but she had broken her good behaviour bond as well. In the District Court, Judge Clegg, referring to her original sentence in the Local Court, wanted to know, 'Who was the optimistic gentleman who thought Miss Miles could keep the peace for twelve months?' When he was told that Mr Gibson, a senior magistrate from the Central Court, had been responsible, he expressed surprise. 'I thought it might have been some new magistrate,' he murmured. Deciding not to take any further action against Bee, he remarked as she left the court, 'I suppose she'll make for the nearest taxi-cab.'[20] The judge knew, as did most people in Sydney, that Bee had a particular preference for taxis.

———

When Bee Miles died in 1973, a cortege of taxi cabs lined the road to Rookwood Cemetery, where her ashes were laid. Given the fact that Bee's most violent encounters and heaviest sentences were a result of her clashes with taxi drivers, this final tribute seems somewhat ironic. Apart from a few notable exceptions, the taxi industry generally held her in contempt. Her disputes with taxi drivers were widely publicised and in time became part of the mythology that grew up around her. In most renderings of Bee in popular culture, she is inextricably linked to taxis.

In 1952 there were 2052 taxi cabs in Sydney,[21] and while most people still relied on trams for transport, taxis were a more comfortable and expedient choice for those who could afford them. Part of the attraction they held for Bee was her belief that she could legally ride in a cab without paying a fare. Her logic went something like this. If a cab was stopped, either at a rank or at traffic lights, she could enter it and if she didn't ask to be taken anywhere, she wouldn't have to pay. Instead, she could stay in the cab. If there were passengers already in the cab, and if they didn't object to her presence, then the cab became her workplace. She would convince the passengers to join her in a wager about how many cabs they might see before they reached their destination. Bee, a veteran of the urban transport system, usually won and often paid the passengers' fare. These more congenial interactions were generally without incident. The cause of most of the disputes between Bee and taxi drivers occurred when they refused to take her as a paying customer. Their objections were almost always concerned with her appearance. 'I object to the state of this woman's attire,' one driver told the police as a justification for refusing Bee's fare.[22] Other drivers told the police they would have to have their cabs fumigated if Bee sat in their vehicles. The words were cruel, but the actions that often accompanied them were inhumane.

On 30 December 1950 a crowd of more than 200 people gathered in a back lane near Central Station as an incensed taxi driver threw buckets of cold water over his passenger, who sat crying in the back seat. Watching with the crowd were several detectives and uniformed police from nearby CIB headquarters. Even though water was cascading down her face, the woman refused to leave the cab. By now the crowd was growing larger and included several journalists, who, while the driver was away refilling his bucket, proceeded to interview the woman, still sitting in the taxi. Bee told them that she had hired the cab in Martin Place to take her to Chatswood, but the driver had taken her to the nearest police station instead. Because she was a paying customer, the police had refused to act, so the driver had driven her to Central Lane, where he proceeded to pour buckets of water all over her.

Bee showed journalists and the crowd a piece of clothing with a ten-shilling note pinned to it, as evidence of her intention to pay the driver, who in the meantime, having refilled his bucket, returned and continued to throw water into the cab. By now the crowd had grown so large that it blocked the surrounding streets. Finally, the detectives intervened, and the taxi drove away with Bee still in the back seat accompanied by the police. At her request she was driven to the Department of Transport so she could make a formal complaint. In the company of the detectives she paid the driver the two-shilling fare. At the Department of Transport she was referred back to the police. The department told journalists that this was the third time Bee had made a complaint about drivers hosing her or throwing water on her. The police later said they could take no action because Bee had paid her fare. There appeared to be no inclination to charge the taxi driver.[23]

Two years later the *Macleay Argus* published what they considered to be yet another humorous anecdote about Bee. Like most rural newspapers, they had a weekly round-up of news from 'the city', and Bee was a regular topic. This time they described an undated incident where she had tried to hire a cab and the driver had declined the fare. Bee, however, was already in the cab and had refused to leave. The frustrated driver had called his employer. 'Along came the boss with a bit of help. One chap held Bee's arms while another put the business end of a hose down her blouse, someone turned on the tap, and in a few seconds, a cold stream of water went squirting on its merry way.' They continued to restrain her until she started to cry.[24]

As if this wasn't humiliating enough, more sinister acts were to follow. In 1955 Bee was in crowded Park Street in the city when she was seen getting out of a taxi to retrieve her eyeshade, which had fallen on the ground. Witnesses saw her trying to re-enter the cab and then a moment later she was lying unconscious, blood streaming from a large gash to her head. Despite protests from the crowd, which by now had grown so large that it was blocking traffic, the attending policeman interviewed the taxi driver 'as Bea lay bleeding at his feet'. Bee was taken to Sydney Hospital by ambulance. There is no record of a charge against the taxi driver.[25]

Not all relationships with taxis were hostile. No longer able to jump rattlers as she had done in her youth, Bee famously engaged drivers to take her on long trips across country during the 1950s. In 1955 she hired Sylvia Markham, Sydney's first female driver, to take her to Perth and back. The purpose of the trip was to collect new wildflower specimens for the Sydney Herbarium. It took Markham and her co-driver nineteen days to cross the country—one of the longest trips by taxi ever undertaken in Australia. Bee paid a shilling a mile, tearing off notes pinned to her coat, a habit she had developed in her itinerant travels in the 1930s to avoid being arrested for vagrancy. There were similar trips by taxi to Broken Hill, Adelaide and Tasmania. These epic journeys served several purposes. They fed Bee's appetite for movement, while providing comfort and safety at the same time. They allowed her the opportunity to once more experience the places she had traversed so often in her younger days—the landscapes she loved. And they allowed her to pursue her goal of finding a new Australian plant to bring back to the Royal Botanic Gardens—a quest she was never able to fulfil. But these well-publicised events also convinced taxi drivers that Bee had significant financial resources, and some would appear at the family's department store, where her brothers were still the managers, demanding to be compensated for fictitious fares. Even other cab drivers acknowledged this was a scam.[26] But Bee's penurious position had not changed. She used money that accumulated when she was in gaol to fund her trips. Otherwise, most of her money went into state revenue from the increasing number of fines the courts imposed on her.

———

The 1950s are often viewed as a period of conformity, where order and respectability were linked as civic virtues. But no society is homogenous, and in every mainstream there are undercurrents that move against the flow. A group known as the Sydney Libertarians— predominantly university educated and intellectual—emerged in the 1950s to claim their inheritance from the bohemians of the 1920s and the anarchist movements of the 1930s. They opposed 'censorship, authoritarianism and moralism' and embraced free thought and sexual freedom. They conducted their acts of intellectual dissent and philosophical inquiry in a selection of former bohemian pubs and cafes or private parties, rarely disturbing the flow of mainstream life.[27]

In contrast emerging subcultures of working-class youth, like Bodgies and Widgies, with their distinctive dress style, long hair and habit of gathering in public places, fed into a broader moral panic about falling community standards. Public anxiety was in turn fed by sensational media reports about gangs of teenagers engaging in violence, bad language and illicit sex—and resulted in draconian responses by police to contain street disorder. At the same time legislators moved quickly to ban comic books, which were seen as having a negative influence on the behaviour of the nation's adolescents.[28]

Although philosophically Bee would have had much in common with the Libertarians, she never identified with them and, like the Bodgies, her disruptions were far more overt. Throughout the

1950s she was increasingly viewed by police as a threat to public order, and there were times when this view was justified. Bee's habit of jumping into cars and demanding to be taken to her desired destination would have been disturbing, if not frightening, for some people—though whether it was illegal is debatable. Equally, the way she walked into the middle of traffic to hail cars, forcing drivers to swerve around her, was at times dangerous and reckless, though this had been ruled as legal by an appeals judge.

But in most cases the charges were petty and were to do with her appearance. 'She was without shoes and stockings and her manner was offensive to me' was a familiar statement by arresting officers. 'Her dress was above her knee,' one policeman claimed, as reason for arresting Bee when she was touting for business as a recitalist on a busy corner opposite the Town Hall.[29] In another incident police at Darlinghurst Police Station were in the process of charging Bee for offensive behaviour when one of her admirers put his arm around her and kissed her. The police response was to charge her again, as well as her companion. At different times she was charged with poking out her tongue at a driver, sleeping in a bandstand and calling a taxi driver a mug. One of the most dubious arrests occurred when Bee was asleep in a garden bed in Elizabeth Street. The police removed her blankets and then charged her with offensive behaviour because, they claimed, her 'bloomers' were exposed. She was fined £5.[30]

———

In a decade that was increasingly prosperous, neat and streamlined, and in which femininity was synonymous with 'glamour and charm', Bee was the anomaly.[31] She was large and untidy and was often without shoes. She wore men's coats and a tennis visor. She was a highly visible, irregular and contrary female presence. Perhaps the contrast between accepted standards of femininity and Bee's appearance was most vividly illustrated on the occasion when she was arrested in Rowe Street. Of all the casualties of the great wrecking ball of progress that ploughed through Sydney in the 1960s and 1970s—and there were many—the destruction of Rowe Street was one of greatest. More like an alleyway than a street, it ran between the larger thoroughfares of Pitt and Castlereagh. The small shops that lined each side of this tiny oasis were an eclectic mixture of haute couture, avant garde furnishings and second-hand chic. Shoppers could browse for hand-painted silk fabrics, Japanese lampshades, tiny ceramic buttons and intricate handmade jewellery. The Nontanda Gallery featured modern European paint-ings, attracting artists and students, and the espresso coffee shops became the haunt of the Libertarians. Girls with perfect posture could be seen entering the ballet school, while Madam Lamont the milliner fitted her latest exclusive creations on the heads of Sydney's wealthiest socialites. People didn't hurry down Rowe Street, they sauntered. Women wore their clothes with style and confidence, stopping in the middle of the street to chat, to look and to be seen. But one warm day in January 1956 the patrons of Rowe Street had their usual reverie interrupted by the sound of stampeding feet. A large, yet remarkably agile Bee Miles was running down its length, her big overcoat billowing out behind her like a sail and her tennis visor flapping up and down as she ran. Behind her was an extremely angry taxi driver, waving and shouting expletives. Elegant shoppers jumped out of the way as Bee hurtled past and dived into a barber shop. She stood for a moment, staring defi-antly at the startled barber, and then darted into his toilet. By now people had started to gather at the shop door, the window displays and the espresso coffee abandoned. A policeman, then another, pushed their way inside until the small barber shop was crowded with people all shouting their advice. The hapless barber was still trying to plead with Bee to come out. But the cubicle was silent. Then they heard a click. Bee had locked herself in. By now there were so many police and onlookers that the crowd overflowed onto Rowe Street. Everyone was shouting. The police wanted to shoulder the door but the barber insisted they come up with a better plan. He went across to the chemist in search of a stink bomb but all he could find was a bottle of ammonia and a pad, which he showed to the crowd. They all watched him as he placed it under the door. Again nothing happened. Then someone suggested a fan, which he put next to the pad, but the fumes blew back onto the barber and the police and sent them spluttering to the other side of the shop. Giggling could be heard coming from the cubicle. After an hour or so a big-framed sergeant stepped forward and shouldered the door. Bee came out quietly and was escorted down Rowe Street by a large contingent of police. The elegant shoppers returned to their reverie and the barber had his picture taken for the paper.[32] Bee would later claim that the driver had punched and kicked her trying to extract £10 from her. She was charged and found guilty and fined £20.

———

The police's general perception of Bee was that she was mentally unstable, but more than likely there was some vindictiveness on their part as well. Bee's comments when being arrested—such as 'get away you fool', 'do not exceed your duty', 'wretched liar', 'big gasbag' or 'you are drunk with power and you are a homosexual'— would have affronted many a member of the constabulary. The claim that 'only a woman with loose morals would marry a police-man', which she would shout as she was being dragged into a police car, wouldn't have helped the relationship either. These phrases, when repeated in court as evidence of her offensive behaviour, were regularly circulated in newspaper articles, usually syndicated, so they were reproduced across the country. They tended to make Bee seem more in control than the police, espe-cially when she won appeals.

Then in 1956, in a provocative move, Bee published a two-page article in *Weekend*, a popular tabloid, entitled 'The Cops and Me'.

In it she listed some of ways the police had harassed her over the years:

> Every kindergarten tot in Sydney knows that when a 'demon' or a copper is getting low on his quota of arrests he goes looking for a drunk, a deadbeat, a street-woman or Bee Miles, who is none of these things . . . If there's one thing the coppers can't stand, it's a person who doesn't conform to convention and yet stays within the law. That's ME. And there are SIX reasons why the cops get at me: 1. They cannot make me leave the city. 2. They cannot get me on a criminal charge. 3. They cannot get me on a vice charge. 4. They cannot get me on a drunk charge. 5. They cannot 'vag' me. I have a small private income so I'm not a vagrant. 6. They cannot get an honest doctor to declare me insane.[33]

This list, which Bee also circulated as a press release to journalists during court hearings, was basically correct. Most of Bee's charges were limited to offensive behaviour. She was never arrested for serious crimes. In the 1950s, thanks to the publication of her court defences, her receipt of a private income from her father's estate was well known and prevented her being charged with vagrancy. She was largely abstinent so avoided arrest for drunk and disorderly. She knew that an offensive behaviour charge often carried connotations of prostitution, though she had no record of soliciting. 'It is very offensive to be on this charge as if I were a woman who solicited men in the street for immoral purposes,' she once complained to a magistrate. The magistrate, with the improbable name of Mr Pickup, assured her that 'no one would think that of you, Beatrice'.[34] But in Bee's mind, and no doubt in the minds of many arresting police, there remained a link between the visible presence of women in the street, immorality and disorder.

By the mid-1950s Bee was so exasperated by the repeated charge of 'offensive behaviour' that she challenged members of the judiciary to come to the Domain 'and define it, then debate it'.[35] In doing so she drew upon a long-standing rationalist tradition of public debate. Her father was known for his 'mordant wit and ruthless logic' in Sunday afternoon sessions at the Domain and at the Trades Hall and had frequently challenged church leaders to public debates in his younger days. Unsurprisingly, no member of the bench came forward to take up Bee's challenge. Instead, she took the debate to them, using the courtroom as a forum to argue her case and propagate her ideas.

———

It was inside the confines of the courtroom that Bee used her talents as a performer and her rhetorical skills to her best advantage. She was not always successful—in fact in most cases, the charges were proved against her—but the courtroom gave her an opportunity to promulgate her views about the fallibility of the justice system and the dishonesty of the police. She was acutely aware that the journalists present in court would be reporting the proceedings, so she came prepared, often supplying printed statements of her speeches to the court. In an era before the concept of the 'sound bite' Bee was able to circulate her most fundamental ideas through pithy aphorisms such as 'When constituted authority comes into conflict with the unauthorised person, believe the unauthorised person,' a phrase that continued to be republished years after her death.

In the decade after the Second World War, Bee's demeanour in court was one of cultivated indifference. She would play patience in the vestibule, casually ask strangers for a cigarette, whistle, sing or lecture waiting police witnesses on the inequities of the justice system. But in the dock her persona would change. She was sharp and eager for debate. Although she later claimed that she always represented herself in court, she used lawyers on multiple occasions. In the 1930s she was sometimes represented by the charming and erudite James Meagher, an Irish-born solicitor, classicist and protégé of James Joyce when they both lived in Paris. In Sydney his practice was in Liverpool Street and his client list ranged from the infamous brothel keeper Tilly Devine to the writer D'Arcy Niland. Meagher was a regular patron of Pakie's and honorary solicitor for the Fellowship of Australian Authors. He was involved in local theatre and literary groups, and published a translation of Ovid's *The Art of Love*. Like Bee, his performances in court were famously flamboyant.[36] But, by the 1950s, the quality of Bee's legal defence declined somewhat when she chose the services of Harold Munro more frequently. Like Meagher, Munro was a well-known solicitor but for a very different set of reasons. Described as the 'legal father confessor to the "other half of Sydney citizenry"', he was regularly reported in the papers on charges that varied from receiving stolen goods to bribing police, all of which he fought successfully.[37] In the 1950s he added to his legal work by staging nude reviews. Like Meagher, he also represented Tilly Devine in a famous case where she was accused of shooting her second husband. He was eventually struck off in 1966, but prior to that represented Bee for twenty years. His defences were rarely successful, and during hearings Bee would sit behind him reading a book—though she would sometimes appeal if found guilty. In the Appeals Courts she often had more luck, particularly when she represented herself.

Newspaper journalists tended to be dispatched to rounds for the lesser courts as a punishment or because they were new to the paper. The cases they covered there rarely resulted in major articles. But when Bee came to court—particularly if she was representing herself—everything changed. Bee was good copy and journalists knew they were more likely to get their story into the pages of the next edition.[38] Bee knew it too and often made their jobs easier by issuing press releases or her latest manifesto. Providing her own statement was also a way of ensuring that their reporting was accurate. 'Newspapers,' she once observed, 'are not on the whole a reliable source of information. They are too inclined to give us what we want instead of what we ought to have. They omit words and sentences and so distort what has been said or transpired.'[39]

Court officials were on alert as well, aware that Bee would often ignore the strict spatial boundaries within the room. This became an increasing problem as she grew older and deafer and would insist on leaving the dock and approaching the magistrate's bench. On occasion she would even try to use the magistrate's door to enter the court. When eventually redirected back to her seat, she would typically refuse to rise for the magistrate, quoting obscure clauses from laws governing court behaviour. She usually gave her address as NFPA—no fixed place of abode—and her profession as a 'student'—of either Shakespeare or Swift, or sometimes 'of life' itself. During court proceedings she would conduct lengthy cross-examinations, pausing every now and then to make sure the court stenographer had recorded all the testimony. Taking careful notes, she would occasionally look up from her writing to call a witness a liar.

Bee knew and understood the power of language. She retained a great affection for Australian vernacular, but when she used formal English, she chose her words with precision. If the charges concerned insulting language against the police, she would argue that they were technically accurate and not obscene. For instance, she pleaded guilty without protest to the charge of calling a police sergeant 'a dirty big greasy pig', when he arrested her for being a nuisance at Sydney Hospital, even though she had gone there for treatment for an injury.[40] But if she disagreed with the charge then she would argue against it: 'I am a reasonably well-educated woman and I object to having those adjectives ascribed to me. I don't swear in terms of coprophilic sex.' Multiple newspapers that reprinted the story explained the term to their readers as 'an abnormal interest in filth'. As her solicitor Harold Munro had once argued (unsuccessfully), 'Although she was insulting, she used delicate words.'[41]

The court hearings also provided an opportunity for Bee to complain about the violence she endured from taxi drivers and, sometimes, police. Answering charges regarding property damage to cabs, Bee would assert that her actions were in defence against drivers who punched or kicked her. If they physically assaulted her, she would use her considerable weight to lean against the open car door and bend the hinges back, sometimes snapping them. At other times she complained that the police had put her in a headlock during arrests. These accusations were largely ignored by magistrates, who tended to focus on the evidence before them of damaged doors and loss of earnings. The fact that drivers did physically assault her was witnessed on several occasions, but never seemed to be addressed directly by the courts. It was an echo of similar claims she had made against her father twenty years before, when he had beaten her in his office before multiple witnesses and the magistrate had chosen to fine her for offensive behaviour instead.

Drivers continually argued that the main reason they refused to take Bee as a paying passenger was because they considered her appearance offensive. 'Her distinctive but unfashionable frocking' as one journalist described it, adding that 'soap and water seem a bit scarce at Bee's domicile when she has one'.[42] From time to time magistrates agreed, claiming that she was a 'disgrace'. One told her angrily in 1946 before a packed courtroom: 'You have been fast going downhill in recent years … you are high … you need a wash.'[43] Another magistrate told the court, in slightly more compassionate terms, 'It's a pity something can't be done about this woman. She is here almost every day and every day she is dirtier.'[44] In the face of these humiliating attacks, Bee was defiant. 'I'm not dirty,' she told the magistrate. But she also understood that, in order to prove that she was not offensive and that she had a legal right to hire a taxi, and in the face of widespread assumptions about her uncleanliness, she would need to provide hard evidence, which is exactly what she did.

In 1950 she was again in court on a charge of offensive behaviour, having refused to leave a cab she had hired in Martin Place. The court was told that the taxi driver, whom Bee referred to continuously as 'that wretched liar', had refused her fare, complaining to the police: 'This woman is filthy. I want her ejected from my cab.' The attending policeman, Constable Moore, agreed and had told Bee in polite but equally direct terms, 'Madam you are no condition to ride in any public vehicle,' to which Bee responded, 'To hell with you, you fool.' As Bee entered the witness box, she handed the magistrate a document. It was a signed statement from Dobson's Turkish Bathhouse certifying that Bee had been attending the baths there six days a week for many years. Was it a Turkish bath or a normal bath, the police prosecutor wanted to know. 'I have an honest hot bath six days a week,' Bee told him, adding that on Sundays, when Dobson's was closed, she had a bath at Sydney Hospital.[45] 'Which laundry do you patronise?' the prosecutor asked. Bee answered easily. 'I wash my clothes at Dobson's every day and dry them on the boiler while I am having a bath.' When the prosecutor suggested she was antisocial, she addressed the court: 'Listen to him,' she exclaimed. 'I am not antisocial. I am only anti the existing social order.'[46] Turning to the magistrate, she summed up her case:

> The constable mistakes shabbiness for dirtiness. I am a very shabby woman but I am clean. An ignorant person may say: 'Get away. You're dirty. You stink.' That is his way of deriding his mental and moral superior. The constable has charged me with offensive behaviour but in his statement he has alleged only that I was in an offensive state and that I used offensive language to him, neither of which is true.

Despite her certificate, her detailed responses and her technical arguments, the magistrate believed the constable's evidence and fined her £2. Adding to the insult was a further £1 fine for witness expenses, which Bee refused to pay on principle, opting to go to gaol instead.[47] Not prepared to let the matter rest, she appealed the sentence, arguing successfully that as the taxi was not in motion when she entered it, she had a right to hire it as a paying customer. The judge upheld her appeal but fined her £1 for telling the arresting officer, Constable Moore, he was 'a fool'. She did not refute the charge.[48]

As well as the ignominy of having to defend her personal hygiene, Bee often had to argue about her sanity—it was something she'd been doing since the age of seventeen. Responding to a comment by a magistrate that she 'was not right in the head', she argued calmly, 'I am quite rational. I know what I was doing. I was seeking a lift in a car.'[49] The questions around her sanity continued across the decade. Magistrates often commented that she should be in another place besides the courts for treatment. But there was no other place. A medical report requested by the court in 1957 stated that she 'was sane but had high nuisance value'. Finally, it seemed, she had a definitive diagnosis about her mental state, something the hospitals had been unable to produce during the entirety of her past admissions. It also confirmed the sixth point in her manifesto: 'They can't get an honest doctor to declare me insane', a statement she continued to circulate to journalists. In court the magistrate noted that 'there would be wild outcry from any mental hospital to which she was sent'. So he sentenced her to three months' gaol instead.[50]

———

Despite her courtroom bravado and her occasional wins, Bee's defences were no match for the entrenched attitude of a court system that rarely disputed the testimony put forward by the police. This in turn reaffirmed Bee's belief that, because police testimony was sometimes false or misleading, it was irrational for magistrates to base their judgements on it. The police, she maintained, were 'practised liars' and the judges were not 'clairvoyants'. It was an opinion she continued to share with the courts and the media at every opportunity.

Because Bee's activities were concentrated on a small geographical area—usually the city centre—she tended to appear before the same magistrates. Two magistrates in particular, Mr Blackmore and Mr Gibson, dealt with her on a regular basis. At times they both showed humour and compassion when Bee came before them. Although they rarely dismissed the charges, they often allowed her time to pay, or placed her on a good behaviour bond, knowing that she would be unable to abide by its conditions. But as the 1950s progressed their patience began to wear thin, and their frustration became more obvious. Time to pay was granted less frequently, which meant she was sent to gaol more often. If the magistrates' impatience was growing, the escalating violence, arrests and court appearances were taking their toll on Bee as well.

In 1956 a reporter claimed that Bee 'had embarrassed a lot of people' when she burst into tears during a hearing. 'She'd gone feminine,' the journalist complained, and was the 'victim of vanity'. Court attendees had been expecting 'a few moments of hilarity', when Bee appeared before Magistrate Gibson, charged with having removed the keys from a stationary taxi and throwing them into the roadway. After the police gave evidence, Bee requested permission to make a statement. 'He [the driver] was rude to me . . . he said he was going to take me to the carwash and have me hosed down . . . he said he'd have to have his cab fumigated now I'd been in it. I'm a clean healthy woman and it was tit for tat.' She was sobbing. The magistrate fined her £5 and refused time to pay. Observers in the court were heard to mutter that she'd 'lost her sting'.[51]

The frequency of Bee's court appearances escalated dramatically during the 1950s. In 1950 she had 98 convictions, but by 1964 the number would rise to 200 with over 300 court appearances.[52] Her relationship with the police had become increasingly antagonistic and magistrates were clearly frustrated by her constant appearances before them. Prosecutors felt she was 'wasn't what she used to be'; magistrates began to describe her as a pest and a menace; while the newspapers used more pejorative terms, like 'weather-beaten', 'seedy-looking', 'haggard', 'wicked giantess' or 'virago'. Over the years the fines she paid contributed an enormous amount to state revenue and they were getting larger, ranging from £5 to £25, while her income remained the same. This meant that increasingly she was choosing to serve time due to an inability to pay. Sometimes she was in the cells for up to ten days before she even came to court because she couldn't raise bail. The days were gone when people would rush forward to pay for her release. By the late 1950s she was less likely to have a choice. In 1957 she was sentenced to three months' hard labour and then a further six months in 1958. She was, she conceded to a magistrate, losing her charm.

14

Love and the Nation

'I am lonely for three reasons:
1   I am a truth speaker and a truth thinker and I prefer and
    have to fly alone.
2   I cannot endure the priggery, cadery, snobbery, smuggery,
    hypocrisy, lies, flattery, jealousy, envy, pretence, conven-
    tional thought, behaviour and speech and affected and
    artificial behaviour upon which society high and low is
    based.
3   Because I have been in gaol more times than I can count.'

Bee Miles, 'Dictionary by a Bitch', p. 17

The history of modernity's triumphs and failures is built into
the architecture of Australian cities. The Sydney Harbour
Bridge, with its long, clean curve of steel, invited visitors through
its gateway and into the delights and pleasures of its metropolis.
A landmark of modern engineering, the bridge straddled the harbour's
massive expanse as a testament to the young nation's progress and
confidence in its future. At the city's southern extremities lay the
manifestations of modernity's other abiding obsession—contain-
ment: the infectious diseases hospital with its leprosarium, the lock
hospital, the Aboriginal Reserve and the prison. These structures,

out of sight and, for most people, out of mind, invited no one into their midst. They were deliberately placed beyond the public gaze.

———

The long trip out to the State Reformatory for Women at Long Bay was a familiar one. Bee had taken it many times before. Usually her stays were short—around ten days. But in the late 1950s, with her court appearances increasing and the magistrates' tolerance declining in equal measure, she was facing much longer stretches; until in 1958, she was sentenced to six months. This was the longest sentence she had ever faced. She had been charged with maliciously damaging a taxi. What the court never heard, or chose to ignore, was that the driver had kicked her up against an oncoming car, which almost killed her.[1]

In previous years she would have been brought to prison by the Number 948 tram—a dedicated transport service that ran between a siding inside Darlinghurst Police Station and Long Bay. Prisoners were escorted from the courts via a subway. Painted in drab brown or olive, with the words 'No Passengers' printed in large letters above its headlight, its single car contained six cells, each holding up to an equal number of prisoners. Two cells were reserved for women. There were no windows on the cell side and the compartments were dark and cramped. It was here that Bee would have sat on her many long and lonely journeys out to Long Bay; the only tram rides that didn't require tickets. By the late 1950s the Number 948 had gone the way of the rest of the tram network and the famous black mariahs—police vans—had taken its place.

Bee had spent much of her life in buildings with grand facades. Ashfield Castle, her grandparents' home, was a Gothic Revival mansion with vaulted ceilings and high balconies that looked over expansive lawns and manicured gardens. The institutions she had been placed in during her twenties were elaborate colonial buildings situated on generous grounds. The Reformatory was yet another structure built on a grand scale, with its imposing Gothic sandstone gates set amongst the sandhills and low-lying scrub. Once she arrived at the prison and passed through its gates, the architecture that surrounded her was of a different kind. Immediately upon entry she would have been taken to the fumigation room just inside the gates, to be stripped of her clothing and 'cleansed'.

The terminology was important. The Reformatory, when it was established in 1908, was designed to be a moral hospital, where some prisoners could be 'cured' through specially developed programs consisting of physical exercise, gradings, rewards and, most important, restricted associations: separation from individual prisoners who were deemed beyond reform.[2] Prison authorities liked to describe this as 'the prevention of contamination of hopeful cases'. Many of these concepts were borrowed from psychiatric practice in the late nineteenth and early twentieth centuries. And, as in a hospital, the head warder, was called 'the matron'. After cleansing, Bee would have been given a medical examination to ensure she was free of venereal disease and then issued with a prison uniform, which didn't seem to change much over the decades she was frequenting Long Bay. It consisted of a striped dress and apron or pinafore with a cap.

One of the Reformatory's most prominent architectural features was the reception area—a large circular glass building. It was here that individual prisoners would sit amongst the decorously placed indoor plants and be interviewed by members of the Ladies Committee of the Prisoners' Aid Society. They would offer them readings from uplifting texts, advice, guidance and occasionally employment as domestics upon release. The committee was comprised chiefly of wealthy upper-middle class women. Their president was Lady MacCallum, the wife of William Miles' old foe from the Shakespeare Society.

Beyond the glass reception area were four brick wings, containing single cells for each prisoner, which radiated off a main quadrangle.

Behind the cell blocks were two large workshops, where women sewed pillowcases that were used throughout the prison system, as well as in the asylums. There was a large industrial kitchen, where food for the prisoners and official visitors was cooked. Prisoners ate in their cells and meals were conducted in silence to limit the opportunity for association with more intractable inmates. The grounds also included a lock hospital to treat prisoners with venereal disease and a chapel. Along with the other women, Bee would have woken up at 4.30 a.m. when the workday commenced. Work consisted of cleaning, gardening, cooking or needlework. Cleaning included scrubbing the long corridors and verandas on hands and knees, a practice that was still occurring in the 1970s.

Next, and harder to imagine Bee performing, was a regime of vigorous physical exercise based on a Swedish program. This was followed by a cold shower bath—something she would not have welcomed. Bee liked her water extremely hot. Afterwards women could read 'suitable literature' in their cells, which were shut at 4 p.m. It's unknown whether Bee had access to her favourite books: Mencken, Swift and Shakespeare. She would have had them with her when she was arrested—she was never without them. Perhaps they were given back to her as she earned her privileges, a practice that she would have recognised immediately, from the very first prison she entered. As in the asylums, privileges were bestowed or withheld according to a prisoner's attitude to work and adherence to regulations. Demonstrations of industry and decorum could earn a prisoner advancement through their gradings and additional privileges such as better rations and extra reading time. At the heart of the regulatory structure was the goal of developing 'self-control' or restraint amongst a population of refractory but mostly reformable women.[3] Bee would have also been familiar with the classification system, developed in the early twentieth century, and still in place in the 1950s—recidivist, remedial and intractable—like the curable and incurable classifications that were still current within the psychiatric system.[4]

Most prisoners had been sentenced for petty offences, including theft, larceny, offensive language, drunk and disorderly. Others were sentenced for more serious crimes, such as procuring abortions and occasionally murder.[5] Despite the fact that most of these crimes were the result of poverty, newspapers like *Truth* reflected the common perception that most women had committed crimes because they had been corrupted by men, 'for the love of love or some man' or because they were merciless and mercenary and were 'hardened' beyond redemption.[6] Prostitutes had always made up a high percentage of the female prison population but this changed dramatically in the 1930s, when organised crime took control over sexual services and women worked in private dwellings. Arrests and prosecutions declined apart from 'freelancers', who were often older women with less currency. These women, who operated publicly, rather than in designated houses, were targeted by police so regularly that their fines became unaffordable compared to their earnings and they were sent to gaol.[7] In the 1940s and 1950s Bee experienced the same problem as her fines grew far beyond her capacity to pay them. Although the Reformatory was built to house more than 200 prisoners, its population rarely reached more than 100. By the mid-1930s the daily average number of prisoners was 42.

Bee rarely spoke about her stays in prison. She didn't place much value in the remedial powers of the 'moral hospital' and said it was 'a rotten place' that made 'bad men worse and good men bad'. The whole concept of gaol as a method of reform was irrational: 'Magistrates, judges and juries are antisocial because they deliberately and with malice aforethought commit men and women to a system of detention which they know are going to make them worse.'[8] But Bee tolerated it as best she could. She had her own cell, in line with the policy of non-association, and this would have suited her because it allowed her to keep to herself. She felt she was different from the women around her. 'I'm among them, but not of them. I don't use filthy language and I don't encourage the girls who steal big things as some of the prisoners do.'[9] But overall, she was less scathing about her fellow inmates than she was of the more upright citizens outside the prison gates. 'In and out of Long Bay,' she once wrote, 'I have rubbed shoulders with gun molls and murderesses, perjurers, rogues and vagabonds, thieves and urgers, pimps and prostitutes, dead-drunks, dope addicts, plonk-wrecks and ordinary down-and-outs.' But far worse, she claimed, were the 'ulcer-ridden, constipated snobs from the suburbs'.[10] In typical rationalist style, she listed the reasons for her own frequent periods of incarceration:

1 I have behaved rationally and naturally in exact antithesis to conventionality and affectedly in that most conventional and affected of all communities
2 I have lived toughly, dangerously, excitingly, exhilaratingly and simply in exact antithesis to softly, safely, calmly, quietly and conventionally in that most degenerate of all communities
3 Honesty has no protection against superior cunning
4 I don't like taking orders from men I think are my intellectual and moral inferiors
5 The odds against me are 3000 to 1
6 I have no common sense.[11]

Bee was 'in and out' of the Reformatory for nearly 30 years, as well as women's prisons in other cities and smaller lockups through-out rural and remote Australia. Over that time she would have witnessed a gradual deterioration across the prison system. By the late 1950s, when she was serving two of her longest sentences at the Reformatory, the buildings and amenities that had been seen as exemplars of modern efficiency were old and in need of repair. Some of practices that had been in place since the prison opened were also seen as outdated. The Prison Reform Council, influenced by advances in social work, made recommendations that focused on intervention, and during the 1950s a more scientific approach to classifications, including interviews by prison psychologists and IQ tests, was introduced.[12] The genteel conversations with the Ladies from Prisoners' Aid had been replaced by a new regime that would see the introduction of parole officers and welfare workers.

Even though Bee was sentenced to six months in 1958, the longest she served was four-and-a-half months. She must have managed to control her behaviour and became eligible for early release under the parole system, or else, like the psychiatric hospitals, her gaolers were anxious to be rid of her. She seemed to have had a less volatile relationship with the prison staff than she had with the staff in the psychiatric hospitals. The warders, she said, were tough but treated the female prisoners fairly, provided they didn't hit them.

When Bee was released in 1958 she used her accumulated funds to buy a wreath for Brigadier Pearl Mason, a Salvation Army officer and prison welfare worker. 'I was in gaol when Brigadier Mason died,' she told the papers. 'There was genuine sadness in Long Bay for there was scarcely one of us who hadn't been helped by her kindness.' Bee had been delegated to arrange and deliver the wreath of red, yellow and blue flowers—Salvation Army colours. She delivered it by taxi to Mason's grave at Uralla in New England with a card that read 'From the Girls in Long Bay'. It was one of the rare occasions when she expressed solidarity with a group.[13] Nevertheless, it is hard to imagine Bee participating in vigorous Swedish exercise programs, scrubbing floors in a cap and apron, or sitting quietly in a glass conservatory, while one of the ladies read 'suitable' literature to her—unless it was Voltaire or Swift. Besides, there was another piece of writing that was occupying her thoughts—she'd written a new book.

———

In the 1950s Bee's court appearances were so regular it was like she was on a conveyor belt, back and forth between the police, the magistrates and the prison. Journalists knew that when she came to court there would be some theatre, perhaps a mixture of drama and comedy, and some one-liners from Bee that would make good copy. Bee rarely digressed from her set speeches. But there was one day in 1955 when an offhand comment by a prosecutor changed the usual scenario. He had suggested that Bee showed 'degeneracy'. Both the court and the journalists seemed puzzled by Bee's extraordinary reaction. She was seething with anger. 'You don't know what the word degeneracy means,' she screamed.[14] Those in the courtroom watching the exchange probably did know what it meant, but it's unlikely they would have shared Bee's definition.

Like many thinkers and social reformers, particularly in the first half of the twentieth century, Bee adhered to the concept of degeneration—the idea that within the progressive march of modern industrial nations the seeds of racial decline had also been planted. Its cause could be hereditary, environmental or both. This concept provided the framework for many eugenically based interventions in medicine and social welfare, to separate out the fit from the unfit. Bee had been the recipient of this approach during her period of committal in the asylums in the 1920s and, while she was an adherent to the same doctrine of racial decline, the way she measured it was very different.

Unlike the broader understanding of degeneration—that certain groups within society had degenerated from a white, middle-class ideal—Bee believed that degeneration was caused precisely because people conformed to social conventions. In other words, it was propriety in all its manifestations—civil, social and judicial—that caused degeneration. For Bee, social conventions had no validity in the natural world that was an endless cycle of birth, struggle and destruction. The notion of racial progress—that cornerstone of modernity—was false and, in Bee's view antithetical, because modern western society was in a state of irreversible decline. The only hope for progress was a return to Aboriginal sovereignty. Rather than adopting the contemporary policy of assimilation—of 'raising' Indigenous people up to the standards of white society—it was the white races who needed to assimilate to Indigenous culture. The Aboriginal race, she argued, was more intelligent and lived in accordance with natural law. Degeneration became the central argument that ran through her final manuscript 'Dictionary by a Bitch', a book she claimed was so controversial that no one would be game to publish it.

Throughout the 1950s Bee made references to this new work she'd written, and although she never revealed its title, she would circulate extracts through her interviews, occasional newspaper articles and public statements. Unlike her previous manuscripts, this latest work was not a linear story. There is no narrator to guide the reader through the foetid, chaotic world of the asylum or along lonely stretches of remote highway. Instead, it takes the form of a critical treatise spanning science, religion, sexual relations and culture. Its tone is subversive, acerbic and always definitive—appropriate for its structure as a philosophical diction-ary. But it is also a manifesto, and its style owes as much to Bee's rationalist heritage as it does to Mencken, the iconoclastic writer who had the most consistent influence on the development of her critical thinking.

Mencken, according to Bee, rated intellectual courage as 'the rarest virtue' to which she added 'moral courage': the ability to 'speak the truth out loud'.[15] Those who possessed this ability were part of a select group of intellectual geniuses—the 'chosen ones' as Bee described them—who included Socrates, Nietzsche, Swift, Voltaire and, of course, Mencken himself. It was an elitism remi-niscent of Norman Lindsay's artist hero and, like Lindsay, the chosen ones were male. In fact, Lindsay had been a great admirer of Mencken,[16] as was Stephensen, whose short-lived publication *The Australian Mercury,* was a homage to Mencken's long-running journal, *The American Mercury.* In the 'Dictionary' a chosen one is an intellectual who places 'no value on appearances, money, social position, what people think, manners, fashion and most tradition . . . he is discontented intellectually and morally . . . he dislikes rules and regulations'.[17] Bee's intellectual genius had a striking parallel with her definition of a 'true Bohemian'.

The 'Dictionary' included a long list of all the beliefs and practices that Bee believed were spurious and indicative of humanity's decline. Chiropractors, card readers and psychics were dismissed as 'balderdash', while suicide and infanticide were defined as logical practices. God ('I can't see him—he doesn't exist') and the Immaculate Conception ('a physical impossibility') were irrational concepts as was illegitimacy. Some of her ideas would have resonance for 21st-century readers, such as establishing an Australian republic and a trading relationship with Japan, but in post-war Australia, with many former prisoners of war still traumatised by their experiences, this would have caused a reaction. And that was the central aim of the 'Dictionary'. Bee was utilising Mencken's methods to challenge conventional thought, but she also borrowed heavily from the style her father and Stephensen had used in *The Publicist*—deliberate provocation, although her focus was different. While they had obsessed about race and politics, Bee's target was relationships between men and women, or more precisely, their failure.

Under the heading marriage, Bee listed fifteen reasons that the institution was bound to fail. It was impossible, according to Bee, for men and women to be in a satisfying marriage for more than five years because most people didn't understand eroticism. To support her claim, she drew upon the work of two sexologists, Havelock Ellis and Norman Haire. Havelock Ellis had been extremely influential in identifying and describing various types of sexual identity in the early part of the century and co-wrote the first textbook on homosexuality. He wrote prolifically and eloquently and one of his most groundbreaking works was the multi-volume *Studies in the Psychology of Sex*, which had a profound influence on Bee. Norman Haire was a leading physician, sexologist and rationalist and, like Ellis, was a proponent of various elements of eugenics. He had a lucrative practice in London in the 1930s and had famously performed the Steinach procedure on the poet W.B. Yeats to increase both his vitality and virility. Concerned about the rise of

Nazism, he returned to Australia and set up his practice but also immersed himself in bohemian Sydney. Theatrical and flamboyant with a talent for performance, in Australia he used a range of media to provide public education about sexual health and sexual behaviour in a period when people struggled to find correct information in an accessible form. He wrote a regular column for the magazine *Woman* and gave a series of radio talks that caused major controversy and outraged religious groups and politicians because of the frankness of his subject matter.[18] He was a frequent visitor to the Burley Griffin community at Castlecrag and was a close friend of Bernard Hesling. It is unclear whether Bee knew him personally, though they would have moved in similar circles, but she read his work.

Bee's treatment of the same subject matter was far more abrasive than the sexologists she referred to. Women were 'frigid' not because of post-natal depression or menopause but because of men's lack of sexual ability. 'To be able to mate with the average man, a woman must of necessity be partly homosexual because the average man is half a woman. (He is one-third woman in his everyday life, two-thirds woman when he makes love.)'[19]

While Bee's prose lacked Ellis's eloquence or Haire's wit and flair, it did tap into to the broader anxieties of the post-war period and in particular the maladjustments between women and men whose former roles had been displaced by the upheaval of war. Her comments about the breakdown in relationships after a period of five years might have stemmed from her own experience with the unnamed man she fell so deeply in love with in the 1930s. But they also reflected the divorce rate, which increased by 55 per cent between 1944 and 1947. While this was seen in part because of hasty wartime marriages, there was a broader concern that marriage and social stability required a focus not seen in earlier times. In response there was a prolific growth in marriage guidance counselling and advice literature offering methods to support the readjustment of both men and women to monogamous heterosexual marriage, a mutually satisfying sexual relationship and stable family lives.[20] This was not the model Bee subscribed to and her own advice on marital stability was radically different. Married men should be encouraged to have 'concubines',[21] while 'the youth of the country should behave a little, as the police would say, immorally. It is the golden mean between promiscuity and repression.'[22]

Although Bee spoke and wrote about the importance of sex frequently, it was not the way she lived her own life. In fact, there was something rather puritanical in her personal responses to the idea of sex. While, by her own admission, she had been sexually active in her twenties, by her early thirties she had adopted a life of 'simplicity and virtue'. She found most men sexually repulsive, and the ones she desired she placed deliberately out of reach. Her long cross-country taxi rides were undertaken with the strict condition that there would be no sexual advances by the drivers. Back in Sydney, taxi drivers would sometimes proposition her as a way of getting her out of their cabs. John Beynon, her friend and confidant, thought she was afraid of sex. Meaningful and lasting sexual relationships with men were ideas for Bee rather than a reality.

Men were not the only ones to come under the 'Dictionary's' unrelenting scrutiny, which was scathing about women as well, particularly feminists. In the manuscript, the most fundamental struggles of feminist campaigns from suffrage onwards—the right of women to control their own bodies and to participate equally in the public sphere—were described as antithetical to natural law, even though Bee had argued all her life for the same rights. 'The sexes are not equal as I said before, woman is physically, morally, and intellectually weaker than man. To try and promote equality of the sexes means the destruction of heterosexuality in the world, that's why I loathe feminists.'[23] Within the family the father should be the indisputable authority:

> The father should be the supreme arbiter of the morals of the
> home when his sons and daughters commit faults he should

244

clamp down on them right away, not wait for his wife to do so because a woman is a weak creature whether she likes it or not and will condone faults in her sons and daughters that no strong man will condone.[24]

Like many of the 'Dictionary's' statements, this passage is steeped in contradiction when compared to the reality of Bee's own life, where her rebellion against her father's authority had led to the eventual fracturing of their relationship. Bee had never taken male authority seriously—she had made a career of undermining it at every opportunity: lifesavers, transport inspectors, magistrates, doctors and police had all been subject to her acts of defiance. 'The average man is afraid of strange women,' she would repeatedly insist,[25] nor did she like taking orders from men who were her 'inferiors'. Now she was advocating a return to a model of patriarchal control that she had rejected four decades earlier. It was a similar paradox to feminism. Viewed in a broader context, however, Bee's rejection of feminism was not unusual for women of her generation. Christina Stead, for example, also born in 1902, expressed similar hostility towards organised women's movements, which she saw as alienating men.[26]

All her life, Bee had been attracted to strong, independent women, beginning with her grandmother and later with the women who ran the hotels and boarding houses and had so impressed her in her travels. But there were other women who, at critical junctures, had played a role in her suppression: her schoolmistresses and the nurses in the asylums. She resented the power they had held over her and had rejected their authority. But underneath all this, and running through Bee's manuscripts, is a disdain for weakness—physical, moral and intellectual—which linked her to the same Social Darwinist thinking that influenced her father and so many of his generation and gave rise to the eugenics movement. And it was this movement that governed the way she, as a single woman, had been classified and controlled in asylums and courtrooms for most of her adult life. In the 'Dictionary' it had all come full circle.

In Bee's bleak and ruthlessly pessimistic view, modernity had severely compromised the gender balance necessary for the nation's survival. If men weren't hyper-masculine, they became weak and 'feminine'; if women were awarded equal status, it would further emasculate men, who, biologically, had to be the leaders. Relationships between men and women could not be maintained because of a lack of genuine sexual freedom and because men failed to be superior, and women failed to pretend they were. The only true and consistent love was love of country, because unlike people, 'the country never changed'. In the 'Dictionary' Bee even briefly considered a more benign model of National Socialism as a form of government to instil the kind of patriotism she thought was lacking in modern society.

As with her father and Stephensen, Bee's rhetoric had moved over the decades, though her point of departure was very different. Bee was never formally aligned with the Left or the Right, and the intellectual landscape she had traversed was not concerned with politics—it was a terrain populated by failed relationships, including her own. Instead, she turned to the more elusive concept of love and belonging: something that had been missing from her life since her father rejected her, all those years ago. 'I am not a loveable woman. I am far too cynical and selfish. On the other hand, I am very loving and having no one to love, I love my country.'[27] But even this admission is unconvincing. Bee was too influenced by the notion of individual dissent to fully adopt a nationalist movement that would require conformity. She was, as Stephensen had described her all those years ago 'a committed individualist'. She gestured towards the nationalism of her father as a replacement for what she saw as the failure of human love. But her real commitment, unfailing and uncompromising, was to freedom, a quest that endured throughout her life.

It is difficult to pinpoint exactly when 'Dictionary by a Bitch' was written. Bee's public references to it begin in the 1950s but its content indicates that it was created not long after the war had finished. That means its chronology can be dated to less than a decade after the collapse of Australia First and the round-up and internment of its members, including Pankhurst Walsh and Stephensen. Bee would have read the reports of the Clyne Inquiry and the humiliating accusations of treason made against her father that would have been devastating for his children. She was convinced her own book would be highly controversial as well, but she was determined to see it in print. Somewhat surprisingly for a book that was arguably the least publishable of anything she had written, Bee did come close to finding a publisher.

———

Frank Johnson is often overlooked in the history of Australian publishing, but from the 1920s to the 1960s he provided important support for many Australian writers, poets and artists. His early efforts were bound up, as so many literary figures were, with the Lindsays.[28] Johnson had been a co-creator with Jack Lindsay and Kenneth Slessor of *Vision*—the journal that broke new ground in Australian literature in 1923. After *Vision* folded, Johnson was still determined to be a publisher of Australian literature.[29] He became the poet Christopher Brennan's literary agent and friend, and published Slessor's first book of poetry. Johnson established Macquarie Head Press and Frank Johnson Publishing and, along with poets like Hugh McCrea and Slessor, he published writers like Dulcie Deamer and Lennie Lower, later branching out into music and art through monthly magazine titles. He also had a major financial success with comic books during the 1940s. By then he was a stout, red-faced, whiskey-drinking extrovert, who could be found most days at the Plaza Hotel at Wynyard, next door to Peapes, drinking with his close friend, the adventure writer Ion Idriess.[30] He was described as tall and handsome, though Norman Lindsay once remarked that he had a head like a coconut.[31] Bee would have known Frank from the 1920s, but she also had a friendship of sorts with the editor of his music magazine *Tempo*: Merv Acheson, the jazz saxophonist and associate of many of Sydney's criminal underworld. Like Bee, Merv had been in prison, though on the more serious charge of shooting a man in the leg in a nightclub, and they also shared the same lawyer—the dubious Harold Munro. When she wrote to Frank about her book, it was from her own cell at Long Bay.

At some stage, before Bee submitted the manuscript to Johnson, she'd given it to Syd Deamer, well-respected and influential editor of many Australian newspapers. At the time Deamer was writing 'Column 8', a section of the *Sydney Morning Herald* he'd created. (The image of the 'granny' that headed the column for years was said to be based on Deamer.) Apparently, the version of 'Dictionary by a Bitch' Bee had given him was a collection of different bits of paper with the text scrawled in pencil. Despite its presentation, Deamer thought it was worth pursuing but claimed he couldn't get Bee to concentrate.[32]

In prison Bee had little else to do but concentrate. She had begun writing to Frank in March 1958, at the start of her six-month sentence. Although it's not clear when she submitted the manuscript, it was probably before she was in custody. The letters refer to proofreading issues and the cover design rather than publication submission. She wanted the book cover to be very plain—black with gold letters and asked him to take particular care with the spelling of her name 'Bee and *not* Bea'. She had changed the title to 'In Brief', a signature phrase used by Mencken in his essays. Her letters discussed potential reviewers and which newspapers might give her a favourable review, including *Truth* and the *Australasian Post*. But she also provided a list of international publications she wanted it sent to, including the *Baltimore Sun*, the *Manchester Guardian*, the *New York Times* and the *London Times*. 'I don't care for admiration and respect,' she told him. 'But I do like the praise and approval of my superiors and two of them, at least live in that country [England]: Aldous Huxley and Bertrand Russell.'[33] She wrote to Frank regularly, each time adding further instructions about where to distribute any profits from sales—the bulk of which was to be divided up for the female children of relatives on her mother's side living in Queensland. Each time she wrote, she asked him to send her a letter. 'Since I've been coming here for 30 years, I have had only one letter. A letter is a godsend.'[34] Apart from the book there was little else to discuss 'since we do nothing in gaol, there is nothing to tell you'.[35] The Swedish exercise program must have ceased.

In July Frank finally wrote back. Rather sheepishly, he told her that he'd been unable to raise the capital for the book. Publishing costs, he explained, would run to £1800 and the book would need to be sold for 17 shillings and 6 pence. At this stage he didn't have a 'financier' to put up the money. He would, he promised, continue to seek a financial backer for the project and, if he secured one, he 'would certainly go ahead with the publication'.[36]

Johnson died two years later in 1960 but Bee continued to look for a publisher. In 1961 *The Bulletin* reported that Bee had brought a copy of 'In Brief' to their office. The selections they published were different from the original manuscript and far more sanitised, which suggests she had rewritten parts of it to make it more publishable.[37] She had also sent a copy to an American publisher. When neither of these avenues proved fruitful, she placed the following advertisement in the *Sydney Morning Herald*: 'Wanted. Publisher for Bee Miles MS. Most forthright destructive criticism ever written—20-pound deposit.'[38] Despite the generous payment on offer, there don't appear to have been any takers.

The book might not have been published in its entirety, but its contents kept reappearing in newspapers throughout the 1960s and 1970s, in interviews and articles and regular features like the *Sydney Morning Herald*'s 'Sayings of the Week'. In 1965 it told its readers that, according to Bee, 'the sort of men who get married are almost without exception commonplace, womanly, illiterate, and unintelligent'.[39] 'Human young,' Bee's 'Dictionary' told *Herald* readers in 1968, 'are the stupidest of all young. They take ten years learning just to wash, feed, talk and dress themselves.'[40] In 1970 *The Sun* quoted the passage that began this chapter, though the references to loneliness and gaol had been removed. In 1985 this version was included in Stephen Murray-Smith's *Dictionary of Australian Quotations*, and again in 1990 when the Macquarie Dictionary produced a similar volume.[41] In one way or another, albeit in increasingly sanitised excerpts, Bee's 'Dictionary' was being published.

There are some interesting parallels between Bee's last manuscript and the experience of William Chidley half a century before her. Though the contents of Chidley's *The Answer* and Bee's 'Dictionary' were very different, they both saw themselves as sex reformers who had a solution to modernity's discontents and they both wanted to reach mass audiences. At the turn of the century Chidley's book had been considered obscene by the authorities but not necessarily by the public who read it. Yet he was arrested and re-arrested on offensive behaviour charges and eventually died in Callan Park, where he had been committed on numerous occasions. Extracts from his publication, which so offended the police, were used by Havelock Ellis in his *Studies in the Psychology of Sex*, the work that had such a strong influence on Bee. In the late 1960s, when the concept of sexual freedom was far less shocking, excerpts from Bee's manuscript didn't raise many eyebrows. But ten years earlier, when she was writing it and enduring so much police harassment, she might have worried that she could suffer the same fate as Chidley and end her days back in the asylum. As it turned out, this wasn't such a fanciful thought, though it was her actions rather than her words that brought her under the scrutiny of psychiatrists for one last time.

15

To Sleep: Perchance
to Dream

'I can prove I'm not insane. I cannot for the life of me prove
I'm sane.'

Bee Miles, radio interview, circa 1970

If the country was in inexorable decline according to Bee, her own
health was not faring well either. Apart from ongoing problems
with arthritis, she was increasingly incontinent. Recollections of Bee
from the late 1950s and early 1960s mention occasional sightings of
her urinating in alleyways, which is how she was arrested in 1959
and returned to the place where her long journey had started—the
Reception House at Darlinghurst.

Initially, Bee had been sent to the State Reformatory for Women
at Long Bay, less than a year after being released in 1958. While
she was there something happened to cause the prison psychiatrist,
Dr John McGeorge, to send her to Darlinghurst for observation.
Her only comment was that 'they did not treat [me] well at Long
Bay'. McGeorge was the first consulting psychiatrist to be appointed
by the Department of Justice as part of the prison system's movement
towards a more scientific approach to prisoner management. A lawyer

as well as a psychiatrist, McGeorge carried out individual assessments and recommended treatment regimes.[1] Bee knew him. Just two years before this latest arrest she had claimed in court that McGeorge 'wouldn't put me in [an asylum], he's on my side'.[2] This suggests that she had been sent to him for assessment on numerous occasions. This time McGeorge had in fact 'put her in'; and the receiving doctors at Darlinghurst appeared to be less on her side than ever.

The brief reports from two psychiatrists who examined Bee, as required under the Act, both agreed that she had a 'gross personality disorder'. Dr Ewan Grey, who had been in practice since the 1920s, reported that he had known Bee for many years and that she had suffered 'a cerebral disease' that had 'so interfered with her conduct and behaviour as to make her live a more or less derelict existence'. Dr Fischer, on the other hand, didn't appear interested in any causal relationships and was clearly affronted by his patient's behaviour, deciding that Bee was 'abusive, arrogant and impossible to deal with'. After two days she was transferred to Gladesville Mental Hospital.[3]

It must have been a difficult journey as Bee retraced the path that had taken her to the gates of Gladesville Hospital in 1923— 36 years before. On her arrival she was given a full examination and despite her incontinence and hypertension, the report noted that Bee's physical health was reasonable. Although she was nearly sixty, her hair was still brown and her face was full. Her bodily condition was described as 'good', though she bore the scars from numerous injuries and operations, and she had scratch marks on her arms. The last time her weight had been recorded was in 1933 at Kenmore: she was then around 66 kilograms. By 1959 she had gained another 30 kilograms, bringing her weight up to nearly 100 kilograms. Bee's behaviour was described as 'demanding and potentially violent' and she was given a diagnosis of 'psychopathic personality disorder', though the report noted that she could also be classified as 'eccentric borderline class of paraphrenics',[4] proving once again that the only consistent feature of her many diagnoses over the years was their variation.

In contrast, Bee's behaviour in the ward seemed consistent with her past admissions, dating back to her first stay at Gladesville when she was 21 years old. She was demanding and restless, quoting Shakespeare, ordering the nurses around and calling them 'idiots', and wanting to be the centre of attention. But there were two key differences. She didn't seem to interfere with the other patients as she had done during her previous stays, and she insisted on sleeping on the floor. Although the case notes describe her as revelling in her own intelligence on the ward, she was more reticent when she was faced with an actual test. The psychologist's report, carried out about a week after Bee arrived at Gladesville, is refreshingly different from the highly critical tone often found in the case notes. Dr Hay described the 'tactical skirmish' that took place when Bee was asked to submit to a series of intelligence tests. Initially, she refused to co-operate, only agreeing after the psychologist underwent Bee's test first, made up of 'searching questions of specialised knowledge'. Dr Hay barely managed to pass, but after another set of probing questions on the test's origin and marking system, the patient finally agreed to cooperate, though every now and then she would interrupt proceedings with 'extremely smutty limericks'. She also refused to participate in any maths-related questions, which Dr Hay interpreted as her 'intolerance of failure'. Though the unanswered questions reduced her score, her IQ was still in the 'superior range' of 123 to 128:

> Her vocabulary and range of Information and Comprehension are remarkable and at a very Superior level and there is no apparent impairment in new learning or powers of abstraction. The general test gives a picture of a normal if pig-headed old lady . . . in no way psychotic . . . an intelligent and imaginative person keenly aware of environmental nuances and well able to think along the lines as other people.[5]

The final diagnosis: non-psychotic behavioural disorder. In terms of a psychiatric diagnosis, it added little value.

When the history of these conflicting diagnoses (often seeming to depend on the examining doctor's moral as well as clinical viewpoint) is considered, there is one element over that 36-year period that is common throughout: not for its presence, but for its absence. In each of Bee's presentations, from 1923 to 1959, there is minimal or no attempt to explain her condition in the context of the disease that almost killed her and sparked her long and troubled entanglement with the health and judicial systems. Instead, what the reports share is a phrasebook of condemnation: 'wilful', 'restless', 'impulsive', 'childish', 'arrogant', 'impudent' and 'tearful'—the same words that are often found in descriptions of the chronic phase of encephalitis lethargica.

———

Encephalitis lethargica was an infectious disease with a short lifespan and a very long afterlife. Its period as an epidemic lasted only seven years (1917–1924), followed by an equal number of years of receding risk, before it seemed to disappear as an acute disease. It was first identified in Vienna during the First World War as a type of sleeping sickness. People suffered headaches, nausea, double vision and delirium, and fell into deep sleeps or 'stupors'. Most patients would survive the acute illness but many would not; in the initial stages of the epidemic, the mortality rate in some outbreaks was as high as 50 per cent, but the overall rate was closer to 20. Those who did survive were often left with symptoms resembling those of Parkinson's disease, including tremors, rigid or mask-like features, and restricted movement, which developed over time and varied in severity. Encephalitis lethargica spread through Europe, England, America and the Pacific, reaching Australia in 1919 via an Anzac returning to Tasmania. In the same year, due to its rapid spread across Europe, Australia had declared it a quarantinable disease, but it was not immediately notifiable in most states, which meant that data collection on the rate and geographical reach of the disease was poor. But cases were spreading, particularly on the east coast from Tasmania to Queensland. Within a year of encephalitis lethargica's first appearance in Australia, Bee had contracted it.[6]

While the cause of encephalitis lethargica—the actual pathogen—has never been identified, by 1930 much more was known about this mysterious disease that seemed to arrive without warning, burn a path of destruction and then disappear almost as suddenly as it had first appeared. When compared with diseases such as influenza or tuberculosis, encephalitis lethargica did not cause the same number of deaths, nor was it as contagious. But it was now clear that patients who contracted encephalitis lethargica and survived its acute phase were permanently altered physically and psychologically. This was known as the chronic phase of the disease. Most patients never fully recovered or resumed the life they had known before they became ill. Many degenerated into a state of restricted movement and were confined to institutions, out of public view and awareness, although their confinement was not always immediate. Most encephalitis lethargica sufferers were under 40 years of age, which meant that the afterlife of the disease was long and progressive. Many were children aged between five and eighteen and their symptoms were different again. In the acute stage of the infection children tended to suffer a type of insomnia. They slept heavily during the day and became manic and highly distressed at night, unable to concentrate, irritable, engaging in pranks and at times more destructive behaviours that led to tragic outcomes. While the insomnia gradually abated, changes in character became apparent. Children became impulsive, and occasionally violent, although the violence was usually an immediate response to an impulse, rather than a planned action. Some children displayed an 'elevated libido', the results of which were sometimes serious and always distressing. Previously well-behaved children and young adults became disobedient, aggressive and unable to control their impulses and emotions. For the families, watching these dramatic changes in their children, it was devastating. As specialists observed, there were 'good boys made bad and bad boys made worse' by encephalitis lethargica.[7] Years later, Bee would describe prison in almost identical terms.

One of the most distinctive features of this 'behavioural syndrome' in encephalitis lethargica sufferers was hyperphrenia, or psycho-motor hyperactivity. Encephalitis lethargica sufferers were impelled to move, not necessarily to reach a destination or with any purpose. It was different from a compulsion, where a person is driven to enact something to obtain an outcome. This was movement for move-ment's sake. It could even extend to 'wanderlust', or the impulsion to travel, and some sufferers were reported to have wandered aimlessly around Europe for years. They were also impelled to touch—to handle things and then immediately discard them, moving on to the next source of stimulus.

In Europe, the United Kingdom and North America, the post-encephalitic behaviour of children and young adults was regarded with concern, particularly in the context of broader anxiety about social degeneration within the general population. But there was additional anxiety about the likelihood that these young sufferers were destined for the criminal justice system because of behaviours and urges they couldn't control. Public and medical lobbying finally led to an amendment to England's *Mental Deficiency Act* in 1927, extending the legal category of 'moral imbecile' (individuals with a 'permanent mental defect' who committed crimes because of their impaired moral sense) to people in whom the defect was acquired. This meant that encephalitis lethargica could be considered as a factor in criminal cases. In Europe it was observed that while 'All who had suffered EL with behavioural problems were in danger of criminality', only a small minority faced court because their mis-demeanours were usually handled by the police. 'Female offenders were especially likely to be directed away from the courts to some form of psychiatric care.'[8] This was clearly not the same in Australia, where in Bee's case, the blame was firmly directed at her 'wilfulness' and 'lack of control', and relatively minor offences usually resulted in court hearings.[9]

Elsewhere in the world a variety of treatments and therapies were trialled, including the opening of a Post-Encephalitis Unit at Winchmore Hospital in London to house and treat young people who would otherwise end up in juvenile reformatories. Similar units were established in various European countries, as well as the United States. The results were mixed; while there were improvements in sufferers with milder symptoms, problematic behaviours often returned once patients were released from care or removed by their parents. The treatment of encephalitis lethargica sufferers was not always benign: it could include heavy sedation and later, in both Britain and the United States, frontal lobotomies. Although neither frequent nor widespread, these were practices that continued until the early 1950s.[10] In Nazi Germany, where eugenic theory reached its fullest and most repugnant manifestation, encephalitis lethargica came under the umbrella of diseases that threatened the country's racial destiny. While encephalitis lethargica patients were not necessarily sterilised under the 1933 Law for the Prevention of Offspring with Hereditary Diseases, they were still subject to official scrutiny. In 1939 Hitler, the man whom Bee would later describe in her 'Dictionary' as a military genius greater than Napoleon, authorised doctors to grant 'mercy killings' in cases of incurable disease. Surveys distributed to sanatoria, asylums and rural hospitals contained a list of eligible candidates that included schizophrenics, epileptics, the 'feeble-minded' and encephalitis lethargica sufferers.[11] Meanwhile, in Australia, increased knowledge about encephalitis lethargica did not correspond with changes to legislation or a more enlightened attitude within the criminal justice system. While the increase in policing powers over the first decades of the twentieth century was not in response to the criminal behaviours of encephalitis lethargica sufferers, these amendments were aimed at the vulnerable populations where sufferers were more likely to gravitate.

Bee was seventeen years old when she contracted encephalitis lethargica in 1920—still a relatively unknown disease in Australia, even though it required quarantine. Her symptoms were typical of those being reported around the country at the time: severe headaches, blurred vision and constantly falling into deep sleeps—the acute stage of encephalitis lethargica. When she finally began to recover, it was obvious that her behaviour had changed. And while encephalitis lethargica was initially recorded in her case notes, sometimes by its name and other times as a passing reference, it was never fully explored and appeared to be treated as something distinct from her behaviour. Chisholm Ross, the doctor who had featured so much in Bee's early life, would have had extensive knowledge of her medical history. He had examined her as a private patient, just after she had recovered from the acute stage of encephalitis lethargica, to assess whether she could manage university study. A year later an editorial in the *Medical Journal of Australia* reflected the increasing sense of calamity in the international medical community, as the results of the first studies into the after-effects of encephalitis lethargica in children began to emerge: 'EL has more terrors than the immediate risk of death . . . nothing concerns a nation more than the welfare of its children.'[12]

Chisholm Ross reappeared as one of the examining doctors at the Reception House when Bee was brought there in December 1923 by her father. Six months earlier a detailed review of encephalitis lethargica in Australia had been completed by Dr Charles Hogg, who held a position at Parramatta Mental Hospital, where Bee would eventually be sent in 1927. Hogg would later rise to the position of inspector general and followed Bee's committals with interest. Given the small number of doctors working across the mental hospital system, it is highly unlikely that Chisholm Ross would have been unaware of Hogg's report. His own report on Bee included a detailed account of what happened during the acute stage of her illness but he didn't link it to her current problematic behaviour, which he ascribed to her failure to adhere to parental control and social propriety. She had always been, his report noted, 'erratic and irresponsible'.[13] He based this statement on information provided by William during Bee's first committal and possibly prior to that when he had examined her as a private patient. William wrote long, detailed letters to the Reception House and then to Gladesville Mental Hospital once Bee was transferred there. Aside from describing the current set of behaviours she developed after contracting encephalitis lethargica, William told the doctors he thought Bee had probably always been insane. She had been 'wilful' from childhood but her moods became increasingly 'stormy' in her last two years at school. It was during this period that she started to demonstrate 'a lack of respect for authority', particularly towards her schoolmistresses. But this was also the period that directly followed the anti-conscription campaigns that had consumed William and dominated his family's lives. He had made his children wear the controversial 'No' badges to school and had advised his daughter on the essay she wrote criticising the Gallipoli campaign that caused so much controversy. These were actions and sentiments that would have created hostility and even enmity in her classmates and teachers, and alienated her at school. Bee, raised in rationalist and free-thought traditions, would have held fast to the dictum her father taught her—to reject arbitrary authority. Her teachers found her attitude intolerable and she began to be threatened with expulsion. But William never acknowledged the way in which his beliefs influenced his daughter's behaviour, and just how firmly he had planted the seeds of opposition in her character. Instead, the idea that Bee's adolescent rebellion was a kind of inherent mental illness entered the patient case notes and her medical history despite the fact that, as early as 1925, the superintendent at Gladesville Hospital had stated that Bee's condition was untreatable and that 'the attack of Encephalitis Lethargica in 1920, was to a great extent the causal factor'.[14]

In 1929, when Bee was arrested and taken back to the Reception House, she was again examined by Chisholm Ross. His notes at the time, while not explicitly naming encephalitis lethargica, describe a group of symptoms that would have been recognised as hyperphrenia and part of the encephalitis lethargica behavioural syndrome. 'She is foolish and childish in her outlook . . . She is well known to me as an erratic person, very unstable and given to acts of law breaking without any sense of responsibility . . . and although she does try to control herself, she is not able to succeed.'[15]

It was a similar story in 1933 when Bee was brought back to the Reception House at the request of a very frustrated doctor at Sydney Hospital. It was over the incident where she kept removing patients' bandages, something that could be explained by hyperphrenia—the impulsion to touch and handle objects. Despite being removed by the police several times, she kept returning and repeating the behaviour. The doctor, whose incandescent rage can almost be seen rising from his letter to the Reception House, was one of the few who noted that Bee probably had post-encephalitic syndrome, to which he also added 'congenital moral defect'. In some ways this was an even more damning diagnosis as it carried the inference that Bee was inherently criminally inclined or morally deficient—notions that gave so much fertile ground to eugenic interventions.

Chisholm Ross resigned from his position at the Reception House in 1931. His final years had been controversial and his evidence in one case regarding a patient's mental competence had been found to be unreliable in court. The presiding judge had castigated him severely. Like Bee, he had been labelled 'a menace to the public'. Though he was later cleared by a Medical Board inquiry, it was an inauspicious end to a successful and influential career.[16] He would also be remembered for his prominent role in the repeated committals of William Chidley. Chisholm Ross's replacement at the Reception House was Dr James Rainbow. Like his predecessor, Rainbow was similarly disinclined to link Bee's former illness to her current list of misdemeanours, again focusing on her deviation from the behaviour expected from a woman of her class:

> Unduly elated . . . impulsive, lacking in control and inter-
> feres with . . . other patients. Is garrulous, foolish in speech
> and childish in her ideas . . . restless, talkative, impulsive and
> interfering. Unable to restrain herself from behaviour unfit-
> ting to a woman of her years and education.[17]

But if we examine Bee's behaviour through the prism of encephalitis lethargica and in particular the behavioural syndrome that followed its initial onset, many of the behaviours that brought her to the Reception House again and again were clearly part of her condition. Journalists always described her as being obsessed with transport—a description that has remained—but it wasn't transport that fascinated Bee, it was movement. The behaviour started not long after she recovered from the acute stage of encephalitis lethargica, when she began jumping on and off trains and trams *while* they were moving. After that she progressed to cars—leaping on to the back or sideboard. When that became more difficult, as she aged and sideboards disappeared, she would open car doors and jump inside, issuing drivers with hurried commands to 'drive on'. All the while she was constantly moving around the country, up and down the east and west coasts, covering vast areas, appearing and reappearing in towns and cities across the continent. Then when she was older and less nimble, she would demand, bargain and sometimes plead to be driven around in taxis for hours on end with no destination. These are all actions that point to an overwhelming impulse to be in constant motion.

In the same way, Bee's behaviour in the asylums during her first committal is typical of the characteristics in patients—particularly children—diagnosed with encephalitis lethargica. The sudden shifts from hyperactivity to tearfulness, attention seeking, pranks, exhibitionism, teasing other patients, violence, intense sexual urges: these are all behaviours described with increasing symmetry in observations of encephalitis lethargica patients across the world. But for the doctors and nurses, faithfully recording Bee's behaviour and trying to reconcile it with her obvious intelligence, class and education, the connection to something other than 'wilfulness' was never made. It also sheds a different light on Bee's home life leading up to her committal: the violent outbursts, the over-eating, the impulsive behaviours and the chaos that made life unendurable for everyone around her.

If the doctors failed to explore the connection with encephalitis lethargica, the police and the prosecutors were equally oblivious. At different times Bee was a public woman or a public nuisance: either way her behaviour was deliberately offensive. Magistrates, even if they understood that there was something else driving Bee's behaviour, were reliant on the evidence put before them and Bee's lawyers rarely referred to her history of encephalitis lethargica, with two exceptions. At some stage, between 1927 and 1929, she was charged with stealing books from Dymocks Bookshop. (She later claimed that they were her books and she was retrieving them after someone had sold them to Dymocks without her permission.) Her father claimed that the charges were dismissed when the famous female police inspector Lillian Armfield testified in court that Bee was insane.[18] In 1932 Clive Arnott, her father's solicitor, told a magistrate that 'the young girl contracted a sleeping sickness when she was a child and that affected her mentally'. In that case, the magistrate dismissed the charges, but not before Bee had shouted at her lawyer to 'shut up'.[19] Bee, who could spend hours arguing the most obscure points of law when conducting her own defences, never used her illness to excuse her actions. In fact, she never discussed encephalitis lethargica in her manuscripts or interviews. It was as though it never happened.

But then again, why would she? Admitting that many of her actions were an impulsion caused by an illness and beyond her control would conflict with, and utterly confound, the carefully constructed rationale for her behaviour. It was a rationale that saw her actions, not as the result of a random pathogen, but as a delib-erate campaign of resistance against an irrational system. And there was another problem. The mention of encephalitis lethargica might link Bee to mental illness and to schizophrenia. The idea that acute encephalitis lethargica could cause schizophrenia was a much-debated topic in the growing international literature on the disease throughout the interwar and post-war periods. Bee, who demonstrated a keen interest in contemporary psychological theory, was aware of the pervasiveness of this idea in medical discourse and the conflation of encephalitis lethargica with other psychiatric disorders. In hospital she challenged her doctors about the link, and in private had confided to her friend Bernard Hesling that she thought she had dementia praecox (an earlier term for schizophrenia). But in public, as we have seen, she consistently linked her behaviour to society's sexually repressive attitudes. Subsequent research into the roles of different brain pathways would show that encephalitis lethargica and schizophrenia were not related, but the stigma around the disease as a type of insanity would remain. In a similar way the myth about Bee's mysterious nervous breakdown through 'over study' would persist long after the reality of encephalitis lethargica had faded from public memory.

There are two elements that make Bee's experience of encephalitis lethargica different from other survivors of the disease. One is the fact that she never developed the form of Parkinsonism that made sufferers immobile. She remained physically active and agile right through to middle age. This was extremely rare for encephalitis lethargica sufferers, whose typical fate was described with dramatic effect in Oliver Sacks' memoir *Awakenings* and with such tragic vividness in Paul Foley's comprehensive study *Encephalitis Lethargica: The Mind and Brain Virus*. The second element that distinguishes Bee was her ability to turn her condition into a public performance and a political act of dissent. Her talent as a performer and her commitment to the bohemian philosophy of living life as an art form, allowed her to rationalise her behaviours as giving way to her 'harmless impulses'.

'Whatever I've done—and believe me I've done plenty—' Bee wrote, 'I've done purely and simply for fun and that's the motive of the highly intelligent woman for being unconventional in public—for fun.' If this was her only motivation, then her long history of arrests, committals and imprisonment seems a very high price to pay.

16

None but Fools
Would Keep

'If God really existed it would be necessary to abolish Him.'

Mikhail Bakunin, *God and the State*

Living and working on the street is hard, particularly as the body grows older and more susceptible to disease or vulnerable to assault. Bee believed that her fame provided a form of public protection that kept her safe from random attacks, and to a certain extent it did. She was never robbed and most of the physical injuries she sustained were from assaults by taxi drivers, arrests, traffic accidents or the occasional fight with an overzealous conductress. But there was one occasion, in 1960, when she was attacked without explanation. She had stopped a car on Parramatta Road driven by a 'young man'. When they were approaching Burwood Road she asked to be let off, but the driver kept going. He drove her a further seven kilometres to Rookwood Cemetery, where he proceeded to beat her. She was found in a dazed and confused state at the cemetery gates by a passing truck driver and taken to a nearby hospital by ambulance. In the middle of the doctor's examination Bee asked to be excused and was seen heading for the bathroom with 'several volumes of Shakespeare'. She never returned.[1]

In 1963 Father John Hope suffered a heart attack and, after a period spent recuperating, he decided to resign after nearly forty years at Christ Church St Laurence. It was the end of an era for the parish and for many individuals who had enjoyed Father Hope's protection. The clergy house, where Bee had been sleeping for many years on the laundry floor, was in serious need of renovation. It was obvious that the extensive repair work could not accommodate an ageing tenant, who by now was sleeping early and rising late. And perhaps some of the tolerance that had been extended to Bee under Father Hope's tenure had lessened with his departure and the start of a new regime. It was around this time that Bee started living in a series of rented rooms, first in London Street, Enmore, and later in Weston Street, Dulwich Hill, suburbs a few kilometres from the city's perimeter.

At the same time, the city's centre, the place Bee had known so intimately, was changing all around her. The streets no longer rattled with the sound of trams lumbering up the hill from Circular Quay. Now they shook from the pounding of jack-hammers as so many graceful old buildings were crushed into dust. The bohemian haunts of her youth were all but gone. Pakie had been run over in Elizabeth Street in 1945 and the club's patronage was dwindling each year. Mockbell's, the cafes where people met, argued and played chess in their lunch hours, were long gone and Repin's coffee shops, which had dotted the landscape of her youth, were starting to close, their buildings progressively demolished. The skyline was obscured by a spider's web of cranes, as new concrete structures of unimaginable height climbed ever upwards.

But Bee still made her rounds, carrying her sandwich board onto suburban buses and plying her trade on the steps of the Library or Beberfald's Corner opposite the Town Hall. There were still occasional reports of arrests for fare evasion, but these were rarer now, as were her confrontations with taxis. She'd had a cameo appearance as a character in Dorothy Hewitt's debut novel *Bobbin Up* and her portrait by Alex Robinson had been entered in the Archibald Portrait Prize in 1961, but for the first time in decades she was not in the papers on a weekly basis, though readers still wrote in with stories about Bee climbing into their cars at traffic lights. Around the same time as she was disappearing from the pages of the tabloids, *Tharunka*, the University of New South Wales student newspaper, began featuring her in a regular series of satirical columns as 'Dame Bea Miles', introducing her to a new generation of readers. Then in May 1964, without fanfare or press release, Bee quietly moved into the Little Sisters of the Poor Home for the Aged at Randwick. Even though she was once more in an institution, this time she went willingly.

―――

Bee's life had come full circle. At the age of 62 she found herself living in a shared domestic setting for the first time since she left her family home in Wahroonga. At the Little Sisters of the Poor, where she settled for a warm bed and three meals a day, her days of sleeping on bandstands and church porches were over. After so many years on the street, these small comforts were a luxury. She had an agreement with the nuns that there would be no attempts at religious conversion, though she insisted she would convert some of them to atheism. Her only concession was to agree to wear a holy medal, a gift from the mother superior. She was once more in the care of women—nurses and nuns—but this time it was different. There were no fights or punishments; instead she referred to her carers as 'angels'.

Somewhat ironically this final institutionalisation offered a kind of freedom, particularly from police harassment and the constant threat of imprisonment. Initially, it also removed her from public view, but slowly articles about her new residence began to circulate. Rather than finding their subject by stormwater drains or in parks, journalists now made their appointments through the home's mother superior. Occasionally Bee would demand a fee, which would consist of a half-kilogram of prawns or an outing in a car. During interviews she would repeat quotations from 'In Brief' and other manuscripts, criticise the police and the judicial system, condemn Australia's continuing relationship with the British monarchy and urge the country's youth to be a little reckless. Despite repeated questioning, she remained circumspect about her background and family, yet she was increasingly reflective about other aspects of her past. 'I've led a hard, cruel, good full life,' she would tell reporters. 'The hardness and cruelty have made me frightfully cynical; the goodness and fullness have prevented me from being neurotic.'[2] Some articles claimed their subject had mellowed and was more benevolent, under headings such as 'The New Bee Miles' or 'Bee Miles . . . Calls Off Her Private War', but they still printed her diatribes against 'the average man' and the impossibility of the immaculate conception. This usually invited the question of how such a famously committed atheist could be living in a Catholic nursing home cared for by nuns. The answer, Bee explained repeatedly, and with uncharacteristic patience, was simple. There were not enough atheists in Sydney to have their own dedicated retirement home. Besides, she added, the nuns were incredibly kind to her.

And so it was that Bee's great quest for liberty and her lifelong commitment to resistance came to rest on the back veranda of a suburban nursing home, where she read Dickens and an assortment of encyclopedias. Physical movement, so central to every aspect of her life, had become more challenging. One arm was now so weak that she was unable to dress or bathe without assistance. She attributed this to an assault by a taxi driver several years before. He had twisted her arm with such violence, he'd almost broken it.[3] Her body was racked with arthritis, and she had developed diabetes, though possibly she'd had the condition for a few years without being diagnosed.

Bee had always maintained a Swiftian view of humanity's foibles, but she did have a tolerance and a level of affection for certain individuals. Towards the end of her life, the person who was probably the closest to what might be termed a friend was a taxi driver. John Beynon had been one of the drivers who had accompanied Bee on a long trip across country to Adelaide in the 1950s. But John was also an old song-and-dance man and occasional actor, who drove cabs to supplement his income. Now he arrived every Thursday morning, promptly at 9.30 a.m., to pick Bee up from the nursing home. From Randwick they would travel to the nearby suburb of Maroubra, where Bee would visit the local library and borrow fourteen books, usually a few of her favourite authors, Nietzsche and Voltaire and a mixture of autobiographies. From there they would travel south or west visiting her favourite parks. Occasionally she might take some of the other residents with her for an outing to Manly—returning to the beach where she had created so much spectacle in her youth. Back in the nursing home she would visit residents who were unwell, bringing them sweets or fruit she'd bought on her outings, holding their hands and reading to them. At times she would sit with the dying, keeping a vigil throughout the night alongside the nuns, keenly observing the way they anointed their patients' failing bodies. She had always been attracted to ritual and her many years of living with the Anglo-Catholic priests at Christ Church St Laurence would have given her intimate knowledge of religious practice. But she remained adamant that there was no God or afterlife, and that any suggestion of her own potential conversion was absurd.

Other than her more public displays of benevolence and compassion, Bee's behaviour had not changed. She was still autocratic, demanding and impatient, shouting out orders to all those around her and smoking the occasional cigarette in the chapel. She was disdainful of everyone else's intellect, particularly the nuns, whose lack of intelligence, she contended, was demonstrated by their choice of vocation. 'They don't come interesting,' she said. She described Cardinal Gilroy, the most eminent Catholic in Australia at the time, as having no conversation and claimed he had admitted to her that he wasn't intelligent.[4] Though she never reconciled with her brothers, Bee did resume her connection with her eldest sister, Constance, who came to visit her at the nursing home. 'Here comes my sister,' she would announce, 'and she's an atheist, too.'

In the early 1970s Bee was interviewed for radio and television. On radio her voice conjured up visions of a stage actor from another century: the long, drawn-out vowels, the rhythmic stresses placed carefully and precisely on each word, without a hint of hesitation. She could systematically and mercilessly dismantle conventional society, while making her vitriol sound like poetry. In newspapers she continued to be featured in quotes of the week and trivia quizzes and was included, along with Barry Humphries, in a list of 'prominent Australians', who were asked what they wanted for Christmas. Bee's response: 'A trip round Australia in a lovely big car.'[5]

Despite her television debut, ongoing media interest in Bee was waning. 'Woman's Angle', a feature in *The Sun* newspaper, interviewed her on her views on 'would-be women liberators', and she responded with her usual declaration that women were 'intellectually, physically, and emotionally weaker than men', though, she conceded, 'morally women are stronger'.[6] There was a brief flurry of attention when it was announced that the pope would be visiting the Randwick Home. Journalists wanted to know how Bee would react. 'I suppose I'll go and see him,' she said. 'He's a handsome dog.' This comment seemed to upset her fellow resident, the appropriately named Gladys Bishop, who attempted to correct her. 'She means the Holy Father has handsome beautiful thoughts,' she suggested. 'Shut up, Bishop,' Bee roared. 'I mean he looks handsome. Italy is the mother of handsome men.'[7] She could still be relied on to supply a controversial comment on a popular topic or provide material on a slow news day, but her days of dominating the weekly reporting rounds for the Australian reading public were over.

The final vestiges of her father's legacy were disappearing as well. Peapes Menswear—the last visible emblem of the family's connection with the city's public and commercial life—was sold; its majestic interiors, the signature design of that esoteric and race-obsessed architect Hardy Wilson, were lost to public view, as were its sumptuous furnishings, upholstered by yet another controversial figure—Francis de Groot. Like Bee, Peapes had been strongly identified with Sydney's history, and newspaper articles marking its closure read like obituaries, mourning the loss of another Sydney icon.[8] With the closure of Peapes, William Miles' last links to the cultural and political life of the city were severed as well. Gone were the forays into Sydney's social and cultural life, the chess championships, the sacred and secular concerts, and the Shakespeare performances. Gone too were the political voices: the early embrace of rationalism and the public tirades against organised religion; the Domain speeches, the fervent anti-conscription battles, the socialist contests of the 1920s, the Aboriginal citizenship campaigns of the 1930s and the sad fall into fascism. The curtain had been quietly but deliberately drawn on the past.

Then in 1973 filmmakers James Ricketson and Jan Sharp paid Bee a visit. Over a period of several months, they conducted a series of lengthy interviews, slowly and patiently drawing Bee out about various aspects of her life. In the past Bee's unwavering response when questioned about her early life was cryptic. She would merely say that from the ages of fourteen to twenty-five her life was unendurable. In all the years of probing by reporters she never changed this response. But gradually, as the interviews progressed, she began to talk in detail. The picture that emerged was of a family in crisis. Relationships were hostile, often giving way to violence. For the first time, she spoke publicly about the series of events that had led to her committal, including the beatings, the jealousies and the predatory behaviour. What she didn't mention was the encephalitis lethargica and the role it might have played in turning a hostile family relationship into domestic warfare.

The question is: why did Bee suddenly decide to reveal details that she had guarded so closely for most of her life? Was it because there was no one's reputation left to protect? The family business was sold, and her brothers had retired. They had all had successful marriages—something she had always felt a family scandal might prevent. Or was it because she knew her own life was coming to an end? Ricketson had asked her to participate in a documentary film he was planning with Sharp. Bee was to be driven around in his car, visiting old landmarks and talking about their significance to her story. She readily agreed and asked to visit the storm canal at Rushcutters Bay where she had lived for several months, and Mason's Café on Elizabeth Street where she had dined on curried tongue and peas for nearly twenty years. Her price for her participation—lunch at the David Jones restaurant, where she wanted to order whatever she liked to eat. A couple of weeks later she asked John Beynon to drive her to Ashfield to visit her grandparents' former home, where she had sat in front of the stained-glass window, picking out the notes on the grand piano under her grandmother's watchful eye.

And then she was gone.

Bee died on 3 December 1973, 50 years after her father had taken her to the Reception House at Darlinghurst on that other December day in 1923. The cause of death was a pulmonary embolism and carcinoma of the rectum.

———

Long before her death, Bee had meticulously planned her funeral and cremation. She had received a small share of the Peapes' sale, some of which she gave to the Little Sisters of the Poor and some to her friend John Beynon. The rest she used to pay for her funeral. She ordered a jazz band to play several tunes outside the crematorium, including 'Tie Me Kangaroo Down Sport', 'Waltzing Matilda' and a calypso version of 'Advance Australia Fair'. A ribbon with the words 'One who loves Australia' was to be draped over her coffin, which was to be covered in native wildflowers. She had also supervised her epitaph on the family monument at Rookwood cemetery, where her ashes were to be spread. Appropriately it was a quote from one of her two favourite Shakespeare plays—*Measure for Measure*:

> Reason thus with life:
> If I lose thee, I do lose a thing
> That none but fools would keep;
> A breath thou art,
> Servile to all the skyey influences,
> That dost this habitation,
> Where thou keep'st,
> Hourly afflict.

It was the same scene her parents had performed in 1912 for the Shakespeare Society and a fitting bookend to her father's epitaph on the other side of the same monument. He had chosen Socrates: 'Death is the greatest of all blessings to men.'

The funeral, Bee's final public performance, drew large crowds and was covered extensively in newspapers and on television. Obituaries in all the major papers treated their subject with a respect that had been largely absent in previous decades. No longer 'seedy' or a 'virago', Bee was 'lovable', 'irrepressible' and a 'colourful character'. This is also the period where the term 'eccentric' began to be linked to her name more consistently. On the morning of the funeral, more than 200 people attended a requiem mass at the Little Sisters chapel, where Bee had often sat smoking. Whether this was part of Bee's carefully planning was never confirmed. More people joined the procession out to Rookwood Crematorium, where Bee's coffin was given a police escort, though it's unlikely that this would have been part of Bee's careful arrangements either. People brought flowers, handkerchiefs and anecdotes, which they shared with reporters. John Beynon, Bee's driver and executor of her meagre estate, was one of the pall bearers and afterwards spoke to journalists about a side of Bee that was very different from her public persona. He described her generosity to strangers, her love of animals and distress at any form of cruelty. Bee's brothers, Arthur and John, and her sister Constance were also present but only Constance spoke to the media. During a brief interview, she tried to dismantle the myth that Bee had suffered a nervous breakdown at university, insisting that it was an illness, but giving no other details. Even if she had, it was probably too late. Fact and legend had become too tightly tangled and the story of a young woman unable to handle the rigours of intellectual study prevailed. But by then another rumour was emerging that was to dominate every subsequent story about Bee—her conversion to Catholicism.

The story of the conversion began to circulate on the day of the funeral. People were questioning why Bee was given a requiem mass and why the nuns were taking photos of the coffin during the service. The home's mother superior confirmed that Bee had 'renounced her belief in atheism and received the rites of the Catholic faith'.[9] The reports on how exactly the conversion took place are conflicting. Some sources claim that Bee, in her last moments, called for Father Aub Collins, whom she had known for many years, and asked to be given the last rites. Another version claims that one of the nuns pinned a holy medal on Bee as she was dying and when the priest saw it, he asked Bee if she wanted to convert, to which she agreed.[10] Still another claimed that she always wore a medal of St Mary from when she first entered the home and refused to take it off, which is very different from what Bee had told a reporter a few years before. Her friends and relatives were sceptical, as seemed Alan Gill, the *Sydney Morning Herald* church reporter, who observed: 'The Little Sisters, who say that Bea was converted to Roman Catholicism on her deathbed apparently had better luck than Father John Hope, who declared her an "avowed atheist".'[11]

While it's unlikely that the Catholic faithful would invent a story about their famous resident's conversion, the circumstances under which it occurred are open to speculation. Constance had visited Bee before her death and said she had been moving in and out of consciousness.[12] This was the vulnerable state her father had feared when his own death was imminent. As discussed, he was so concerned that he issued a statement saying that if he recanted his atheism, it would only be because his brain tissue was dissolving. Bee never took the same preventative measures, but up until the night before she died, she was still refusing to be blessed.[13] Another incongruous aspect to the story is the presence of 'Bumper' Farrell at Bee's bedside while she was dying. Farrell, a burly police officer and former football player, was not known for his gentle handling of suspects or prisoners. He'd arrested Bee on numerous occasions during the 1940s and 1950s, and his presence during her last hours remains difficult to fathom. He is said to have 'sat at the end of her bed . . . and held her hand while she abused him'.[14] He also attended her funeral.

———

Bee had always insisted that there was no afterlife, but with every decade that passed after her death, her image continued to be resurrected. Two years after Bee's funeral, *The Coming Out Show*, a new ABC radio program, was launched as part of the International Women's Year. Its unapologetically feminist perspective broke new ground in the way women's issues had been traditionally treated in the media. One of its first programs was a documentary on Bee, produced and presented by Jan Sharp, who had visited Bee along with Ricketson in her last months of life. Dymphna Cusack, Bernard Hesling, Kylie Tennant and George Finey shared their memories of Bee as they knew her in the 1920s: playing the piano at Pakie's, leaping on to the back of Bentley cars, looking glamorous at garden parties or startling in shorts. Sharp's final summation was that Bee was 'a rebel who never developed her own ideas' because she was too influenced by her father. 'She was frozen in the role of the rebellious adolescent daughter as though time had stopped for her in the twenties.'[15] But for a new generation of women this was a very different Bee from the figure they would have seen or read about as they were growing up. This was a woman who broke new ground by breaking rules—she was young, she was radical and she was defiant. When it was announced that the new postage stamps for 1975 were to feature women, *The Bulletin* facetiously claimed that 'the late lamented Bea [sic] Miles was on the list' of candidates.[16]

In 1978 Ricketson placed an advertisement in the *Sydney Morning Herald* asking for 'stories, anecdotes and any information' about Bee. The response was immediate. Two weeks later 'Column 8' reported that Ricketson had been fielding 300 calls a day. The next day the *Sydney Morning Herald*'s own phones rang constantly with people who had more stories to share. While Ricketson was developing a screenplay based on Bee's life, she made her first debut as a fictional character on screen. Dorothy Hewitt played a minor role as a homeless woman in Jim Sharman's film *The Night the Prowler*, based on Patrick White's novella. Though the character was an alcoholic, the greatcoat and tennis visor were unmistakable references to Bee. Then in 1979 Keith Dunstan's book *Ratbags* was published. With a Foreword by Barry Humphries, who also featured in the book, *Ratbags* was a collection of character sketches that included Xavier Herbert, Percy Grainger and Germaine Greer. The chapter on Bee, drawn from newspaper articles, was sympathetic but lacked the depth of Gavin Souter's more nuanced portrait, included in his 1965 book *Sydney*. Dunstan's book sold out in its first week.

Despite Bee's emphatic and repeated rejection of feminism, she was starting to attract the attention of a new generation of feminist scholarship that had begun to emerge in universities across the country—a development Stephensen would have regarded with horror. This had never been part of his vision for a focus on Australian studies in tertiary institutions. In 1980 *Uphill All the Way*, edited by Kay Daniels and Mary Murnane, was published. It was a groundbreaking piece of research that provided a guide to mostly unpublished historical material written by and about Australian women held in public libraries and private archives. Excerpts from two of Bee's manuscripts, 'Advance Australia Fair' and 'For We

Are Young and Free', were included, but not 'Dictionary by a Bitch'. Writing in the *National Times*, Anne Summers described the discovery of Bee's manuscripts in the Mitchell Library as an example of the way new research would 'enable women's history to be included in the so-called general histories of Australia'. A large of photo Bee accompanied the article. After so many years of rejection, her writing—at least in part—was being acknowledged, by the feminists she said she loathed.[17]

Around the same time, writers to the letters section of the *Sydney Morning Herald* began promoting the idea of a statue. The suggestion had come from a contributor named David, who suggested a statue of Bee in the forecourt of the newly renovated Queen Victoria Building opposite the Town Hall. While some writers were suspicious about the sincerity of David's suggestion, the proposal created intense debate about what kind of image the statue should capture and where it should be located. May Phyllis Guest was offended by the photo of Bee that had accompanied David's letter. 'Why put down Bea Miles as a fat old woman . . . Her statue, if taken up seriously, should be sculptured as she was in her heyday, young, strong, athletic and vibrant.'[18] The letter had included the story of Bee swimming out to try to save May's drowning brother at Palm Beach in 1939. Other readers suggested that more suitable candidates should be considered, like the nineteenth-century merchant and philanthropist Mei Quong Tart. After all, one writer argued, what had Bee ever contributed to society?[19] In the end the lord mayor, Doug Sutherland, put an end to the debate declaring that he wouldn't support the idea because 'he believed in the orderly running of the city' and a monument to Bee might encourage people to follow her 'disruptive' lifestyle.[20]

In 1984 Bee took to the stage in a musical entitled *Better Known as Bee*, which was performed at the Q Theatre in Penrith. Co-written by David Mitchell, Ian Dickson and Peter Thornburg with music by Tony Reeves, the musical dramatised the major events in Bee's life through a combination of humour and pathos. The songs and dialogue, drawn directly from Bee's public speeches and interviews, captured her rhetorical style with its use of assonance and rhythm and her love of cataloguing or lists. The portrait that emerged was a mixture of intelligence, humour and irreverence. No doubt Bee would have enjoyed the songs—she had always composed satirical ballads. The musical was a critical success with several productions between its debut and 1992. Some of the scenes and characters were fictional, introduced as plot devices, including the character of Brian Harper (based loosely on Bernard Hesling). In the musical he is Bee's long-time lover who shares her early adventures and then tries unsuccessfully to convince her to lead a more conventional life. In reality they were never romantically involved as Hesling made clear in his 1965 memoir. But as with so many of the myths that evolved about Bee, the fictional Harper became historical fact when he was included in Bee's 1986 entry in the *Australian Dictionary of Biography*, as the long-term love interest she refused to marry.[21] The *Australian Dictionary of Biography* version was republished in the 1988 edition of *200 Australian Women*, one of a number of publishing projects aimed at bringing women's lives into the traditionally male narrative of Australian history. Around the same time, the first dedicated service for homeless women with mental illness was opened in Sydney's Eastern Suburbs. It was a collaboration between the Departments of Housing and Communities and Justice (something Bee might have found ironic). It was named the B Miles Women's Foundation in recognition of Bee's 'strength and determination'.[22] If Bee had lived to experience its services, it might have caused her to acknowledge that feminism had its benefits.

The same year the musical premiered, a first novel by the writer Kate Grenville won *The Australian*/Vogel's Literary Award. Originally titled *Bea's Story*, it was later released as *Lillian's Story*, and was an immediate success, winning a host of literary prizes when it was published two years later. A powerful and lyrical work, it told the story of Lillian, the victim of various forms of abuse by her father when young, who is released after being institutionalised for 40 years. Grenville always acknowledged that, while the novel was inspired by Bee's life, it was a work of creative fiction. Patrick White, whose endorsement appeared on the cover of the first edition, praised Grenville for transforming 'an Australian myth into a dazzling fiction of universal appeal'. As the literary critic Peter Craven noted, White had done the same decades earlier with the nineteenth-century explorer Leichhardt in the novel *Voss*.[23] But White had also grasped the transformation that had occurred in the continuous, elliptical refiguring of Bee's story over time—she had become mythical. In the minds of the reading public and the media, Lillian and Bee would merge—fiction, fact and legend now becoming increasingly indistinguishable.

This entanglement became more evident as the decade gave way to the 1990s and Bee's incarnations, always slightly altered, took on a different shape. The band Ice House released a song about her entitled 'Anything is Possible', with all proceeds donated to charity. We can but speculate as to how Bee might have reacted, given her often-stated aversion to public benevolence. Perhaps she might have quoted her favourite extract from *South Wind* on the evils of charity, or she might have just ignored it. In 1994 news of a film version of *Lillian's Story*, with Ruth Cracknell cast in the lead role, once again evoked a flood of letters to the *Sydney Morning Herald*. There was no attempt to separate fact from fiction as images of Bee cascaded through its pages for weeks: Bee playing patience in the grand vestibules of banks, or on a traffic island in the middle of busy Taylor Square; or emerging majestically from the surf with a knife strapped to each thigh; or cycling down George Street in an evening dress. Under the heading 'Bee's bloomers', there were stories of her sterilising her underwear at Sydney Hospital; or making wagers with bus passengers during their morning commutes to the city.

Not everything was affectionate nostalgia. An enraged correspondent by the name of Mark wrote to the paper claiming, 'I too have memories of Bee Miles. She was an ugly, untidy, aggressive slut of a woman', who had destroyed the livelihood of innocent taxi drivers, flaunted her atheism and cynically taken advantage of charity extended to her by the Little Sisters of the Poor.[24] Predictably his letter produced a raft of correspondence in response. Writers leapt to Bee's defence: 'Don't be unfair to Bee—she was not an alcoholic or a drug taker and was well educated until she had a nervous breakdown.'[25] Others pointed to Bee's 'inner goodness' and respect for and conversion to religious faith. This latter point, underlined by many comments about Bee being in 'heaven' created more controversy. Bill Barlow, related to Bee on her mother's side and a family historian, wrote a lengthy piece that inferred that his relative's deathbed conversion had been performed when she was in an unconscious state: 'Anyone who knew Bee Miles would affirm that she would never, in her normal state of mind, consent to being baptised as suggested by your correspondent. I think it appalling that anyone, during their last moments of life, should be humiliated and harassed by bedside evangelists.'[26]

After six weeks, the letters editor saw the need to draw a line under a debate that created a new momentum with each contribution. 'We've had enough Bee Miles mail to fill an anthology,' the paper noted.

But Bee kept reappearing. As the conservation battles over the proposed development of Bondi Beach and the closure of Luna Park raged in the 1990s, the ghost of Bee was conjured up as a way of demonstrating the significance of each site to Sydney's cultural history. The images of Bee taking a sheep to sunbake on Bondi Beach or swimming with knives were used repeatedly to argue against Bondi's proposed redevelopment. Memories of Bee at Luna Park in the 1930s became a lament for an older Sydney, lost in the push for modernisation.

———

As the twentieth century drew to a close, the New South Wales State Library staged a major exhibition entitled *Eccentrics: A Celebration of Individuals in Society*. 'Sydney,' the Foreword to the exhibition declared, 'has always had a rich history of unusual characters, and it is truly a civil society which can recognise and accommodate this difference and diversity in its midst.'[27] Things had clearly moved on since the library banned Bee from its reading rooms. The exhibition covered the period from white settlement onwards. Bee was featured, along with William Chidley, Arthur Stace, Rosaleen Norton, Dulcie Deamer, Norman Lindsay and Francis De Groot—figures who, by coincidence, had intersected with her own life in various ways. But a more common link between them is tenuous. It's arguable whether Deamer and Lindsay would have seen themselves as eccentric or marginal. Deamer was, in her time, a widely published novelist and successful freelance journalist. Lindsay's artistic vision dominated painters and writers for decades. Although some of his work was subject to censorship, he was at the pinnacle, not the margin, of artistic influence. Neither De Groot nor his supporters thought he was eccentric; nor did the conservative press. When he upset the bridge opening, he was hailed as a hero, and newspapers claimed that Francis would be a popular name for babies born that year.

Rosaleen Norton, on the other hand, was frequently harassed by police and her work branded obscene by authorities. Journalists referred to her as the 'witch of the Cross' and she didn't experience much tolerance during her career. Bee considered Norton a 'silly arse' and would have disputed any philosophical or cultural link between them. If she had ever met Stace, she would have told him that his incessant engraving of 'Eternity' all over Sydney was a waste of time because there was 'no afterlife', although she would have admired his fine copperplate lettering. The one figure Bee might have felt some affinity with was Chidley. She would have supported some of his teachings and disagreed strongly with others, but she would have admired his courage and the way he persevered with his message despite unrelenting police harassment. Even so, it's doubtful that she would have felt that she was aligned with any of the exhibition's other subjects. As a 'truth speaker' Bee had always had to 'fly alone'. And she would never have sat comfortably under the banner of 'eccentric'. It was a term that could provoke anger or tears, depending on the situation. Her reasons for rejecting it lay in the same library's archives. Within the pages of the 'Dictionary', Bee's final work, is a rough pencil sketch. It has a circle in the middle with the words 'average man' in its centre, while three other words, 'eccentricity', 'insanity' and 'imbecile' radiate out from the circle across the page in all directions. Underneath the heading 'Genius Insane' she had written: 'It is of no use putting the grades of man into squares or oblongs. When we say a man is eccentric we mean he is away from one centre or another. There is no centre to a square or oblong. Eccentricity and insanity surround us all.'[28] For Bee, labels and categories, modernity's enduring legacy, were meaningless.

There is a tendency to mythologise our cultural icons according to our needs. They remain as nostalgic representatives of another era that was less conformist and more tolerant of difference. If that era ever really existed in the previous century, it wasn't reflected in judicial or policing practices.

Like all myths and legends, Bee's image continues to shift over time. She is still referenced in stories about eccentric figures or social histories of Sydney, though nowadays she is more likely to appear in a blog about dissident women or a cabaret performance.[29] In all her various renderings as a proto hippy, a rebel, a republican, an early feminist, a victim of patriarchy and even an anarchist, her intellectual strengths and her literary aspirations continue to be submerged by her appearance, her conflicts with taxis and her flamboyant behaviour, under the ubiquitous label of eccentric.

The one eloquent exception can be found in a series of articles written by Gavin Souter. Of all the hundreds of journalists who wrote about Bee throughout her career, Souter was unique in his determination to look beyond her appearance and behaviour and focus on her intellectual strengths, her literary ambitions and her courage to live out her beliefs. In his numerous biographical sketches of Bee during the 1950s and 1960s, he avoided the term eccentric.

Instead, he preferred to describe Bee as a 'character' in the true definition of the word, as someone who made 'a distinctive' impression on her surroundings and in doing so left an indelible mark on those around her:

> Legend insists that we are anti-authoritarian, and so it comes of something of a disappointment to realize that in fact most of us are quite docile. We are circumscribed by regulations . . . and when we are caught stepping out of line we usually go quietly. There are some, however who do not go quietly, who diverge magnificently from the norm and these we celebrate because they help to preserve an illusion which otherwise we should lose entirely. I am thinking . . . particularly of Bee Miles, who never goes quietly . . . One cannot help but be grateful to her for continuing to display that outlaw spirit which has been tamed in the rest of us, if in fact we ever did possess it.[30]

More importantly than how we might describe Bee is what her life tells us about ourselves—about the duality that lies within our national character. We are, as Souter observed, a relatively compliant society. But we also maintain a fascination with those few individuals who 'diverge magnificently from the norm'. Although they sit at the periphery of our vision, there is a quality in their determination, their courage and their commitment that causes us to shift our focus for a moment and to see our world through a different lens. And there is no one in the previous century who held the public's glance and affection for as long as Bee Miles. Despite the best attempts by the custodians of public order to push her to its edges, she kept returning to the centre, each time paying an increasingly heavy price.

Bee's abiding quest to be a published writer was never fully realised. She later reflected that her strengths lay more in oratory than written prose. Fortunately, because of her habit of endlessly quoting herself, we have both. Read sequentially, her writing and her public speech create a remarkable reflection of the twentieth century's cultural history, narrated by a voice that is sometimes profound, often acerbic and always fearless. She was both a product and an observer of a complex and contradictory period, when the inherent tensions within modernity came to threaten the same modern western democracies that created them. She was an unrelenting critic, 'setting the standards' by holding a mirror to contemporary life and finding it wanting, and every now and then turning the reflection on herself:

> Fourteen reasons people dislike me:
> I am cynical, restless, critical, impatient, tactless, excitable, selfish, untidy, inconsiderate, careless, disagreeable, greedy, egotistical, I have forgotten one, lazy.

> Six reasons people like me:
> I am honest, truthful, sincere, forthright, reasonably well educated, very intelligent for a woman, lots of intellectual and moral courage. [I] don't live by fear.[31]

Acknowledgements

My first thanks go to Associate Professor Peter Kirkpatrick who, many years ago, alerted me to Bee's manuscripts in the Mitchell Library and suggested I look at them. Reading them, I was immediately struck by this singular voice, erudite and perspicacious, that spoke to me directly off the page. But I was also aware that these manuscripts were intricately linked to a time and place I knew almost nothing about, even though they were set in the century and the country in which I was born. That realisation led to a PhD where I explored the strange swirl of the twentieth century ideas and events that so influenced Bee's life, her intellectual development and her resistance.

During my doctorial research I had the great fortune to be supervised by that impeccable historian, Professor Alison Bashford. I couldn't have wished for a better guide. In the process of writing the biography I have been equally fortunate. Professor Emeritus Peter Kuch generously commented on early drafts of this book and has continued to encourage me at every stage of its development.

I remain indebted to him. Associate Professor Rob Kaplan kindly shared his own research and his time as he guided me through the complexities of early twentieth century psychiatric practice. Dr Paul Foley patiently led me through the labyrinth of encephalitis lethargica and commented on relevant chapters. Stephensen's biographer, Dr Craig Munro, provided me with perceptive feedback and fascinating discussions and permission to quote from his papers.

Members of the Miles family have been equally generous and encouraging. I am profoundly grateful to them for providing permission to quote from Bee's manuscripts and for their constant encouragement and offers of assistance—in particular, Devon and Dianne Drew, Matthew Miles and Susan Miles, Cathy Drew, the late Annette Lee and Michael Lee, and the late Bill Barlow.

I thank the Librarians of the National and Mitchell Libraries for permission to quote from various manuscripts, as well as the Fryer and Randwick Libraries and the National Archives for research assistance. The archivists at Museums of History NSW have been invaluable and I thank them, along with New South Wales Ministry of Health for permission to quote from Bee's case notes.

I thank James Ricketson for his support and for permission to quote from his interviews with Bee, and David Mitchell for background information on his musical *Better Known as Bee*. I also thank Gavin Souter, surely our greatest writer on Sydney, for permission to quote from his unpublished manuscript and for his recollections.

I thank the many people who wrote to me to share their memories of Bee, some of which appear in this book. I thank the archivists at Abbotsleigh for Bee's school photo and information on her school years. The amazing volunteers—especially Dale Budd—at the Sydney Tramways Museum, who provided me with wonderful photos; and Peter Kingston's estate, which kindly gave permission to use the image of Peter's marvellous tram artwork. I am also grateful to Joseph Waugh at Christ Church St Laurence for providing me with photos and for connecting me with John

Pollard and John Lee, whose memories of Bee painted such clear and vivid word pictures.

During the research and drafting of this book I was ably assisted by Evangelia Ellis who patiently read several versions of the manuscript. I am also grateful to Kirsty McEwan, Dr Elizabeth Barrett, Dr Cathy Marshall, Dr Ian Cameron, Greg Snook and Ariadne Ellis for their helpful comments and careful reading of the manuscript, and for Jean Rhodes for her brilliant photographs. Any errors are mine.

Maria and Louie Armentis kindly opened their beautifully restored home Ambleside for me so I could see the music room. I also thank my friends Yiorgos and Stella for giving me the use of their quiet and beautiful farm, where part of this book was written.

I was fortunate to have Elizabeth Weiss as my publisher at Allen & Unwin, whose wisdom and experience were so beneficial in bringing this work to fruition. Editors Courtney Lick and Susan Keogh were wonderful to work with.

Finally, I would like to thank my ever-patient partner, Yiorgos, for packed lunches, support and encouragement.

List of Bee Miles' Unpublished Manuscripts

Bee Miles, titled variously, 'Prelude to Freedom' and 'Advance Australia Fair', unpublished manuscript, Frank Johnson Papers, Mitchell Library, ML MSS 1214/22, Item 2.

Bee Miles, 'Dictionary by a Bitch', unpublished manuscript, Frank Johnson Papers, Mitchell Library, ML MSS 1214/22, Item 3.

Bee Miles, 'For We Are Young and Free', Frank Johnson Papers, Mitchell Library, ML MSS 1214/22, Item 4.

Bee Miles, 'I Go on a Wild Goose Chase,' unpublished manuscript, Mitchell Library, ML MSS 3225, Item 2.

Bee Miles, 'I Leave in a Hurry', unpublished manuscript, Mitchell Library, ML MSS 3225, Item 1.

Notes

Preface

1   Graham Edwards and Robert Kaplan, 'The Enigma of Bee Miles: Asylum, Anguish, and Encephalitis Lethargica', *Health and History*, vol. 20, no. 1, 2018, pp. 93–119.

Chapter 1: On the Battlements

1   Bill Barlow, *Voyage of the "City of Brisbane" 1862*, Barlow Music, Sydney, 1993.
2   *Illustrated Sydney News*, 3 August 1870.
3   *Empire*, 27 July 1870; E.J. Scartlett, 'Cordner, William John', *Australian Dictionary of Biography*, vol. 3, Melbourne University Press, Melbourne, 1969.
4   *Evening News*, 1 July 1871; 'Theatricals', *Freeman's Journal*, 15 October 1870, p. 7.
5   'Acta Populi', *Freeman's Journal*, 18 August 1910.
6   Bruce Muirden, *The Puzzled Patriots*, Melbourne University Press, Melbourne, 1968; P.R. Stephensen, 'The Death of "John Benauster"', *The Publicist*, February, 1942.
7   Barlow, *Voyage of the "City of Brisbane"*.
8   D. Drew, personal communication.
9   Constance Drew interview with James Ricketson (undated), Mitchell Library Oral History, 535/1–4.
10 Bee Miles correspondence with Bruce Muirden, 22 June 1965, Bruce Muirden Collection, Papers 1942–1968, Fryer Library, University of Queensland, UQFL142, Box 1.
11 Hardy Wilson, C421, Item 55, National Archives of Australia, Canberra.
12 Craig Munro, *Wild Man of Letters: The Story of P.R. Stephensen*, Melbourne University Press, Melbourne, 1984.

13   Constance Drew, interview with James Ricketson.

14   Bee Miles, 'I Leave in a Hurry', unpublished manuscript, Mitchell Library, ML MSS 3225/1, Item 1, p. 32.

15   Constance Drew, interview with James Ricketson.

16   P.R. Stephensen, 'Valedictory Address', 11 January 1942, Stephensen Papers, Mitchell Library, ML MSS 1284, Box 42.

17   Quoted in Ray Dahlitz, *The Secular Who's Who*, R. Dahlitz, Melbourne, p. 59.

18   Bee Miles, 'Dictionary by a Bitch', unpublished manuscript, Frank Johnson Papers, ML MSS 1214/22, Item 3, p. 1.

19   Muirden, *The Puzzled Patriots*, p. 7.

20   Bee Miles interview with James Ricketson, 25 August 1973, Mitchell Library, MLOH, 535/1–4.

21   Ibid.

22   Miles, 'Dictionary by a Bitch', p. 2.

23   Bee Miles, 'The Cops and Me', *Weekend*, 1 December 1956.

24   Verity Burgmann, *Revolutionary Industrial Unionism: The Industrial Workers of the World in Australia*, Cambridge University Press, Melbourne, 1995.

25   Tom Barker was an influential socialist and leading member of the IWW in Sydney at the time of the anti-conscription campaigns. He was the author of an infamous and inflammatory anti-conscription poster and was imprisoned on sedition charges after the IWW was declared unlawful. Twelve other IWW members were imprisoned on charges of treason and suspected arson. For more detail see Ian Turner, *Sydney's Burning*, Alpha Books, Sydney, 1969.

26   Anti Conscription League Minute Books, 1916–17, Mitchell Library, ML A1523.

27   Lewis Rodd, *A Gentle Shipwreck*, Thomas Nelson, Melbourne, 1975.

28   Ian Turner, *Sydney's Burning: An Australian Political Conspiracy*, Alpha Books, Sydney, 1969.

29   Anti Conscription Papers, Mitchell Library, F91/49–51.

30   Anti Conscription League Minute Books, 4 March 1917.

31   William Hughes, 'To the Women of Australia', cited in Joan Beaumont, *Broken Nation: Australians in the Great War*, Allen & Unwin, Sydney, 2014, p. 238; Robin Archer et al (eds), *The Conscription Conflict and the Great War*, Monash University Press, Melbourne, 2016.

32   Michelle Cavanagh, *Margaret Holmes: Life and Times of an Australian Peace Campaigner*, New Holland, Sydney, 2006.

33   Bee Miles, 'I Go on a Wild Goose Chase,' unpublished manuscript, Mitchell Library, ML MSS 3225, Item 2, pp. 15–16.

34   Ibid.

35   Abbotsleigh School Report, April 1911–September 1919, Abbotsleigh Archives.

36   Anti Conscription League Minute Books. Imperial Federation was a movement, mainly driven by politicians and intellectuals, to create a constitutional-based alliance between the different countries of the British Empire. It gained more currency between Federation and World War One. For a detailed discussion see Carolyn Holbrook, 'Anzac, Empire and War: Australian Nationalism and the Campaign for Imperial Federation', *Australian Historical Studies*, vol. 52, no. 1, 2021, pp. 42–62.

37   'Miles on Tour', *The Socialist*, 13 September 1918.

38   Annual Report of the Rationalist Association, 1919.

39 *Sydney Morning Herald*, 18 April 1916.
40 These were the well-publicised sedition cases of Ernie Judd and Percival (Jack) Brookfield. Both men had fractious relationships with the Labor Party and stood for election several times during their careers. They spoke regularly at the Domain, along with William, and the charges resulted from their speeches, which were deemed 'likely to encourage disloyalty' and for making statements 'likely to prejudice recruitment'. 'The Judd Case' *Sydney Morning Herald*, 5 November 1918, p. 4; *Armidale Chronicle*, 25 January 1919; *Australian Worker*, 27 June 1918; *Barrier Miner*, 17 August 1917.
41 *Australian Worker*, 20 November 1919, p. 11.

Chapter 2: Trouble on the North Shore Line

1 Gladesville Hospital, MHNSW – StAC:NRS 5030 [3/6965] T180.
2 Bee Miles interview with James Ricketson, 25 August 1973, Mitchell Library, MLOH, 535/1–4.
3 Gladesville Hospital, MHNSW – StAC:NRS 5030 [3/6965] T180.
4 Bruce Scates, 'A Democratic Rendezvous: The Bookshops of Radical Sydney', in Terry Irving and Rowan Cahill (eds), *Radical Sydney: Places, Portraits and Unruly Episodes*, University of New South Wales Press, Sydney, 2010; Rob Watts, 'Beyond Nature and Nurture: Eugenics in Twentieth-Century Australian History', *Australian Journal of Politics and History*, vol. 40, no. 3, 1994, pp. 318–34.
5 Katie Holmes, '"Spinsters Indispensable": Feminists, Single Women and the Critique of Marriage, 1890–1920', *Australian Historical Studies*, vol. 29, no. 110, 1998, p. 76.
6 Hazel Rowley, *Christina Stead*, Minerva Press, Melbourne, 1994, p. 53. In fact, William and David Stead were both members of the Rationalist Society at the same time.
7 Gavin Souter, 'The Outlaw', unpublished manuscript, 1956, copy in possession of the author.
8 Graham Edwards and Robert Kaplan, 'The Enigma of Bee Miles: Asylum, Anguish, and Encephalitis Lethargica', *Health and History*, vol. 20, no. 1, 2018, pp. 93–119.
9 Bill Barlow, personal communication.
10 Gladesville Hospital, MHNSW – StAC:NRS 5030 [3/6965] T180.
11 Constance Drew interview with James Ricketson (undated), Mitchell Library Oral History, 535/1–4.
12 Edwards and Kaplan, 'The Enigma of Bee Miles'.
13 W.J. Miles correspondence, Gladesville Hospital, MHNSW – StAC:NRS 5030 [3/6965] T180.
14 Ibid.
15 Dora Birtles, personal communication.
16 Miles, interview with James Ricketson.
17 Gladesville Hospital, MHNSW – StAC:NRS 5030 [3/6965] T180.
18 Ibid.
19 Ibid.
20 Ibid.
21 Miles, interview with James Ricketson.

22 Edward Barrett Moulton-Barrett famously disinherited his children when they married, including his daughter, the poet Elizabeth Barrett Browning.

23 Miles, interview with James Ricketson.

24 Gladesville Hospital, MHNSW – StAC:NRS 5030 [3/6965] T180.

25 Ibid.

26 Ibid.

27 Ibid.

28 Miles, interview with James Ricketson.

29 'A Sydney Effort at Democratic Unity', *The Socialist*, 22 March 1918.

30 'Mr Miles and the RPA', *The Socialist*, 30 January 1920, p. 1.

31 *Australian Worker*, 20 November 1919.

32 *Sydney Morning Herald*, 18 December 1923.

33 Gladesville Hospital, MHNSW – StAC:NRS 5030 [3/6965] T180.

34 Bee Miles, 'Advance Australia Fair', unpublished manuscript, Frank Johnson Papers, Mitchell Library, ML MSS 1214/22, Item 2, pp. 1–2.

35 *NSW Police Gazette*, 2 March 1927.

Chapter 3: Wanting in Control

1 Stephen Garton, *Medicine and Madness*, New South Wales University Press, Sydney, 1988; Martin Crotty et al., *A Race for Place: Eugenics, Darwinism and Social Thought and Practice in Australia*, University of Newcastle, Newcastle, NSW, 2000.

2 Stephen Garton, '"Sound Minds and Healthy Bodies": Reconsidering Eugenics in Australia, 1914–1940', *Australian Historical Studies*, vol. 26, no. 103, 1994; Michael Roe, *Nine Australian Progressives: Vitalism in Bourgeois Thought 1890–1960*, University of Queensland Press, Brisbane, 1984.

3 Garton, *Medicine and Madness*, p. 59.

4 Ross Jones, 'The Master Potter and the Rejected Pots: Eugenic Legislation in Victoria, 1918–1939', *Australian Historical Studies*, vol. 30, no. 113, 1999, pp. 319–42.

5 Rosemary Berreen, 'Illegitimacy and Feeble-Mindedness in Early Twentieth-Century NSW', in Jane Long et al. (eds), *Forging Identities: Bodies Gender and Feminist History*, University of Western Australia, Perth, 1997, pp. 202–25.

6 See for example the *Report of the Committee of Inquiry into the Feeble-Minded*, 1914, which claimed: 'In Australia, few outside the medical profession realise the gravity of the problem of the mentally deficient, its relation to crime and to multiplication of the unfit in the community', cited in Garton, *Medicine and Madness*, p. 59.

7 John Murphy, *A Decent Provision: Australian Welfare Policy 1870–1949*, Ashgate, Farnham, 2011, pp. 102–5; Renate Howe and Shurlee Swain, 'Saving the Child and Punishing the Mother: Single Mothers and the State 1912–1942', *Journal of Australian Studies*, no. 37, 1993, pp. 31–46.

8 Ann M. Mitchell, 'Mackellar, Sir Charles Kinnaird (1844–1926)', *Australian Dictionary of Biography*, vol. 10, Melbourne University Press, Melbourne, 1986; Mark Finnane, 'From Dangerous Lunatic to Human Rights? The Law and Mental Illness in Australia', in Catherine Coleborne and Dolly McKinnon (eds), *Madness in Australia: Histories, Heritage and the Asylum*, University of Queensland Press, Brisbane, 2003, pp. 23–33; Grant Rodwell, '"Persons of Lax Morality": Temperance, Eugenics and Education in Australia, 1900–1930', *Journal of Australian Studies*, no. 64, 2000, pp. 62–74.

9 Diane B. Paul, 'Social Darwinism and Eugenics' in Jonathon Hodge and Gregory Radick (eds), *The Cambridge Companion to Darwin*, Cambridge, UK, 2003, pp. 214–39.

10 Garton, *Medicine and Madness*, p. 87.

11 Graham Edwards and Robert Kaplan, 'The Enigma of Bee Miles: Asylum, Anguish, and Encephalitis Lethargica', *Health and History*, vol. 20, no. 1, 2018, pp. 93–119.

12 Gladesville Hospital, MHNSW – StAC:NRS 5030 [3/6965] T180.

13 Jill Julius Matthews, *Good and Mad Women: The Historical Construction of Women in Twentieth-Century Australia*, Allen & Unwin, Sydney, 1984, pp. 145–57.

14 Bee Miles, 'Advance Australia Fair', unpublished manuscript, Frank Johnson Papers, Mitchell Library, ML MSS 1214/22, Item 2, pp. 1–2.

15 Constance Backhouse, '"Her Protests Were Unavailing"; Australian Legal Understandings of Rape, Consent and Sexuality in the Roaring Twenties', *Journal of Australian Studies*, no. 64, 2000, pp. 14–33.

16 Frank Bongiorno, *The Sex Lives of Australians*, Black Inc., Melbourne, 2015, p. 91.

17 Lisa Featherstone, *Let's Talk About Sex: Histories of Sexuality in Australia from Federation to the Pill*, Cambridge Scholars Press, Newcastle, NSW, 2011, p. 58.

18 Bee Miles interview with James Ricketson, 25 August 1973, Mitchell Library, MLOH, 535/1–4.

19 Ibid.

20 Ibid., p. 1.

21 Ibid., p. 8.

22 Ibid., p. 4.

23 Ibid., p. 8.

24 Garton, *Medicine and Madness*, p. 147.

25 Michelle Henning, '"Don't Touch Me (I'm Electric)": On Gender and Sensation in Modernity', in Jane Aruthers and Jean Grimshaw (eds), *Women's Bodies, Discipline and Transgression*, Cassell, London, 1999, p. 22.

26 Matthews, *Good and Mad Women*, p. 114; Garton, *Medicine and Madness*, p. 137.

27 Garton, *Medicine and Madness*, p. 138.

28 Miles, 'Advance Australia Fair', p. 11.

29 Ibid., p. 24.

30 Elaine Showalter, 'Victorian Women and Insanity', in Andrew Scull (ed.), *Madhouses, Mad-Doctors and Madmen: The Social History of Psychiatry in the Victorian Era*, The Althone Press, London, 1981, p. 320.

31 A.T. Edwards, *Patients are People*, Currawong Publishing Company, Sydney, 1968, p. 104.

32 Miles, 'Advance Australia Fair', p. 8.

33 Ibid., p. 6.

Chapter 4: Constraint

1 Desley Deacon, *Managing Gender: The State, the New Middle Class and Women Workers 1830–1930*, Oxford University Press, Melbourne, 1989.

2 Gail Griffith, 'The Feminist Club of NSW 1914–1970: A History of Feminist Politics in Decline', *Hecate*, vol. 14, no. 8, 1988, pp. 56–67.

3 Jackie C. Horne, 'Empire Hysteria and the Healthy Girl', *Women's Studies*, vol. 33, no. 3, 2004, pp. 255–6; Catriona Elder, 'The Question of the Unmarried: Some Meanings

of Being Single in Australia in the 1920s and 1930s', *Australian Feminist Studies*, no. 18, Summer 1993, pp. 153–4; Stephen Garton, 'Freud and the Psychiatrists: The Australian Debate 1900 to 1940', in Brian Head and James Walter (eds), *Intellectual Movements and Australian Society*, Oxford University Press, Melbourne, 1988, p. 173.

4 Lisa Featherstone, *Let's Talk About Sex: Histories of Sexuality in Australia from Federation to the Pill*, Cambridge Scholars Press, Newcastle, NSW, 2011, p. 49.

5 A.T. Edwards, *Patients are People*, Currawong Publishing Company, Sydney, 1968, p. 156.

6 This is a reference to the Shakespeare comedy *All's Well That Ends Well* and the character Parolle's speech on the futility of virginity: 'It is not politic in the commonwealth of nature to preserve virginity. Loss of virginity is rational increase, and there was never virgin got till virginity was first lost.'

7 Bee Miles, 'Advance Australia Fair', unpublished manuscript, Frank Johnson Papers, Mitchell Library, ML MSS 1214/22, Item 2, p. 4.

8 Gladesville Hospital, MHNSW – StAC:NRS 5030 [3/6965] T180.

9 Frank Bongiorno, *The Sex Lives of Australians*, Black Inc., Melbourne, 2015, pp. 74–5.

10 Gladesville Hospital, MHNSW – StAC:NRS 5030 [3/6965] T180.

11 Miles, 'Advance Australia Fair', p. 7.

12 Jill Julius Matthews, *Good and Mad Women: The Historical Construction of Women in Twentieth-Century Australia*, Allen & Unwin, Sydney, 1984, p. 118; Ruth Ford, '"Lady Friends and Sexual Deviationists" Lesbians and the Law in Australia, 1920s–1950s' in Diane Kirby (ed.), *Sex, Power and Justice: Historical Perspectives of Law in Australia*, Oxford University Press, Melbourne, 1995, pp. 33–49.

13 Miles, 'Advance Australia Fair', p. 3.

14 Gladesville Hospital, MHNSW – StAC:NRS 5030 [3/6965] T180.

15 'She Rides Bikes and Bumper Bars', *The Arrow*, 1 January 1932, p. 3.

16 Miles, 'I Go on a Wild Goose Chase,' unpublished manuscript, Mitchell Library, ML MSS 3225, Item 2, p. 48.

17 Mark Finnane, 'The Ruly and the Unruly: Isolation and Inclusion in the Management of the Insane', in Carolyn Strange and Alison Bashford (eds), *Isolation: Places and Practices of Exclusion*, Routledge, Milton Park, UK, 2003, p. 96.

18 Miles, 'Advance Australia Fair', p. 9.

19 Ibid., p. 28.

20 Alison Bashford and Carolyn Strange, 'Isolation and Exclusion in the Modern World', in *Isolation: Places and Practices of Exclusion*, p. 4.

21 Stephen Garton, *Medicine and Madness*, New South Wales University Press, Sydney, 1988, p. 27.

22 Stephen Garton, 'Policing the Dangerous Lunatic: Lunacy Incarceration in New South Wales, 1870–1914' in Mark Finnane (ed.), *Policing in Australia: Historical Perspectives*, New South Wales University Press, Sydney, 1987, pp. 74–8. Elsewhere Garton has also noted that the police arrest rates for lunacy rose steadily from 1895 to 1920, differing substantially from other forms of arrest. See Garton, *Medicine and Madness*, p. 48.

23 Mark Finnane, 'Sexuality and Social Order: The State versus Chidley', in Sydney Labour History Group, *What Rough Beast? The State and Social Order in Australia*, Allen & Unwin, Sydney, 1982, pp. 193–219.

24 Gladesville Hospital, MHNSW – StAC:NRS 5030 [3/6965] T180.
25 Miles, 'Advance Australia Fair', p. 28.
26 Ibid., p. 29.
27 Erving Goffman, *Asylums*, Penguin, Harmondsworth, UK, 1971, p. 48.
28 'Brutality in Asylum', *Northern Star*, 17 March 1923.
29 Miles, 'Advance Australia Fair', p. 28.
30 Edwards, *Patients are People*, p. 61.
31 Garton, 'Seeking Refuge: Why Asylum Facilities Might Still be Relevant for Mental Health Care Today', *Health and History*, vol. 11, no. 1, 2009, pp. 25–45; Anne Digby, *Madness, Morality and Medicine: A Study of the York Retreat*, Cambridge University Press, New York, 1985; Andrew Scull, 'Modern Treatment Reconsidered: Some Sociological Comments on an Episode in the History of British Psychiatry', in Andrew Scull (ed.), *Madhouses, Mad-Doctors and Madmen: The Social History of Psychiatry in the Victorian Era*, The Althone Press, London, 1981, pp. 105–18; Garton, *Medicine and Madness*, p. 13; Milton Lewis, *Managing Madness: Psychiatry and Society in Australia, 1788–1980*, AGPS Press, Canberra, 1988.
32 Garton, 'Seeking Refuge'.
33 Edwards, *Patients are People*, p. 18.
34 Miles, 'Advance Australia Fair', p. 22.
35 Death Certificate, Beatrice Miles, 3 December 1973.

Chapter 5: Flight

1 Death Certificate, Maria Louisa Miles, 11 November 1925.
2 'Madhouse Mystery of Beautiful Sydney Girl', *Smith's Weekly*, 19 March 1927, p. 1.
3 'Missing Friend', *Daily Telegraph*, 25 January 1926, p. 9.
4 NSW *Police Gazette*, 27 January 1926, p. 56.
5 Gladesville Hospital, MHNSW – StAC:NRS 5030 [3/6965] T180.
6 Bee Miles, 'Advance Australia Fair', unpublished manuscript, Frank Johnson Papers, Mitchell Library, ML MSS 1214/22, Item 2, p. 30.
7 Ibid., p. 19.
8 Ibid., p. 32.
9 Gavin Souter, 'The Outlaw', unpublished manuscript, 1956, copy in possession of the author.
10 NSW *Police Gazette*, 2 March 1927, p. 117.
11 George Finey, interviewed for the *Coming Out Show*, ABC Radio, 13 December 1975.
12 George Blaikie, *Remember Smith's Weekly*, Rigby, Sydney, 1966.
13 R. Mowatt, 'Letters', *Sydney Morning Herald*, 25 June 1994.
14 'Madhouse Mystery', *Smith's Weekly*.
15 Kenmore Hospital, MHNSW – StAC:NRS-17418-11-447-4789.
16 Ibid.
17 Douglas Stewart, *A Man of Sydney: An Appreciation of Kenneth Slessor*, Nelson, Melbourne, 1977, p. 41.
18 Kenmore Hospital, MHNSW – StAC:NRS-17418-11-447-4789.
19 Gladesville Hospital, MHNSW – StAC:NRS 5030 [3/6965] T180.
20 Kenmore Hospital, MHNSW – StAC:NRS-17418-11-447-4789.

21 Ibid.

22 David Roth, 'Chemical Restraint at Callan Park Hospital for the Insane, Sydney, New South Wales 1877–1920', *Health and History*, vol. 20, no. 1, 2018, pp. 1–27.

23 Stephen Garton, 'The "Tyranny of Doctors": The Citizen's Liberty League in New South Wales, 1920–39', *Australian Historical Studies*, vol. 25, no. 97, 1991, pp. 340–58.

24 'Mental Hospitals Highly Praised', *Sydney Morning Herald*, 6 April 1923.

25 Mark Finnane, 'The Ruly and the Unruly: Isolation and Inclusion in the Management of the Insane', in Carolyn Strange and Alison Bashford (eds), *Isolation: Places and Practices of Exclusion*, Routledge, Milton Park, UK, 2003, p. 92.

26 Miles, 'Advance Australia Fair', p. 15.

27 Garton, 'The Tyranny of Doctors'.

28 Bee Miles, 'Dictionary by a Bitch', unpublished manuscript, Frank Johnson Papers, Mitchell Library, ML MSS 1214/22, Item 3, p. 4.

Chapter 6: Adventures in Bohemia

1 George Blaikie, *Remember Smith's Weekly*, Rigby, Sydney, 1966, p. 237.

2 Bayview House closed in 1946 and the site became the headquarters of W.D. & H.O. Wills Tobacco, a firm Bee was in frequent correspondence with regarding proposals for sponsorship. It then became the site for the offices of Penfolds Wine and is now an Ikea Store.

3 *Truth*, 11 March 1928.

4 The following texts were used for general background on bohemian Sydney: Peter Kirkpatrick, *The Sea Coast of Bohemia*, University of Queensland Press, Brisbane, 1992; Tony Moore, *Dancing with Empty Pockets: Australia's Bohemians*, Murdoch Books, Sydney, 2012; Ray Lindsay, *A Letter from Sydney*, Jester Press, Melbourne, 1983; Philip Lindsay, *I'd Live the Same Life Over*, Hutchinson, London, 1941; Peter Kirkpatrick (ed.), *The Queen of Bohemia: The Autobiography of Dulcie Deamer*, University of Queensland Press, Brisbane, 1998; Jack Lindsay, *The Roaring Twenties*, London: Bodley Head, London, 1960; Claude McKay, *This is the Life*, Angus & Robertson, Sydney, 1961.

5 George Finey, *The Mangle Wheel: My Life*, Kangaroo Press, Sydney, 1981.

6 Tony Moore, *Dancing with Empty Pockets*, pp. 117–143.

7 Jack Lindsay, 'Australian Poetry and Nationalism', *Vision*, vol. 1, 1923, p. 34.

8 Kirkpatrick, *The Sea Coast of Bohemia*, p. 34.

9 *Triad*, vol. 7, no. 9, 1922, p. 68.

10 Louise Lightfoot, 'With the Burley Griffins', unpublished manuscript, Donald Leslie Johnson Papers, National Library of Australia, MS7817.

11 'Beatrice Miles', *The Coming Out Show*, ABC, 13 December 1975.

12 Ibid.

13 Gladesville Hospital, MHNSW – StAC:NRS 5030 [3/6965] T180.

14 Ibid.

15 Ibid.

16 Ibid.

17 Ibid. No record of these reviews has been found, but they could have been sold as paragraphs, which typically omitted the author's name.

18 Ibid.
19 Beverley Kingston, *A History of New South Wales*, Cambridge University Press, Melbourne, 2006.
20 Bernard Hesling, *The Dinkum Pommie*, Ure Smith, Sydney, 1963.
21 Bee Miles, 'I Leave in a Hurry', unpublished manuscript, Mitchell Library, ML MSS 3225, Item 1, p. 39.
22 'Bee's Story', *The Australian Magazine*, 27 April 1996.
23 Hesling, *The Dinkum Pommie*.
24 'Secrets of the Town', *The Sun*, 7 September 1930.
25 Kirkpatrick, *The Sea Coast of Bohemia*, p. 281.
26 Bee Miles, 'I Go on a Wild Goose Chase,' unpublished manuscript, Mitchell Library, ML MSS 3225, Item 2, p. 45.
27 Gavin Souter, 'The Outlaw', unpublished manuscript, 1956, copy in possession of the author.
28 Deamer, *The Golden Decade*.
29 Souter, 'The Outlaw'.
30 'Beatrice Miles', *The Coming Out Show*.
31 Joe Lynch was a black-and-white artist who worked for *Smith's* and other publications. On the night of 14 May 1927 he disappeared off a Mosman ferry, possibly weighed down by bottles of beer he was carrying in his pockets. His death is the subject of his friend Slessor's poem 'Five Bells'.
32 'The Terror of the Bumper Bar', *Arrow*, 1 January 1932.
33 Bee was always extremely careful about libel and rarely identified any of her contemporaries, even those who were close friends like Bernard Hesling.
34 Bee Miles, 'Dictionary by a Bitch', unpublished manuscript, Frank Johnson Papers, Mitchell Library, ML MSS 1214/22, Item 3, p. 10.

Chapter 7: Playing the Game

1 Gavin Souter, 'The Outlaw', unpublished manuscript, 1956, copy in possession of the author.
2 The fine was paid by Leigh Rankin, identified by Bee as 'a friend'.
3 Bee Miles, 'I Leave in a Hurry', unpublished manuscript, Mitchell Library, ML MSS 3225, Item 1, p. 7.
4 Ibid., p. 1.
5 Amy Johnson was the first woman to fly solo from England to Australia in 1930. Her successful career was cut short when her plane crashed into the Thames in 1941. Her body was never recovered.
6 'Women's letter', *The Land*, 11 June 1930.
7 'Secrets of the Town', *Sun*, 27 December 1931.
8 *Sydney Morning Herald*, 14 February 1932.
9 'Bee's Big Adventure', *Sun*, 1 November 1931.
10 'The Terror of the Bumper Bar', *Arrow*, 1 January 1932.
11 'A Highway Woman', *Queensland Times*, 16 July 1929.
12 *Sydney Morning Herald*, 29 January 1932.
13 Bee Miles interview with James Ricketson, 25 August 1973, Mitchell Library, MLOH, 535/1–4.

14 As well as being a senior member of the New Guard, De Groot was a successful manufacturer of interior furnishings. Specialising in Queensland maple, he had been hired to undertake the refurbishment of Peapes' store in 1928.

15 The *Australian Dictionary of Biography* entry for Bee Miles incorrectly identifies this person as Brian Harper.

16 Bee is referring to Mrs Meagher's defence of the African American boxer Tiger Payne. Payne toured Australia several times in the 1920s and 1930s and his flamboyant style created national media interest and controversy.

17 'Pert Melbourne Girl', *Daily News*, 26 April 1933.

18 Bee Miles, 'I Go on a Wild Goose Chase', unpublished manuscript, Mitchell Library, ML MSS 3225, Item 2, p. 53.

19 Miles, 'I Leave in a Hurry', p. 78.

20 'Girl's Pranks in the City', *Herald*, 24 June 1933.

21 Bee later claimed that this was because she had 'indulged in the innocuous amusement of ringing the bell of the dummy of a tram'. Miles, 'I Go on a Wild Goose Chase', p. 30.

22 Ibid.

23 Medical Certificate, Darlinghurst Reception House, 30 August 1933, MHNSW – StAC:NRS 5030 [3/6965] T180.

24 Kenmore Hospital, MHNSW – StAC:NRS-17418-11-447-4789.

25 Miles, 'I Go on a Wild Goose Chase', pp. 33–4.

Chapter 8: Jumping the Rattler

1 Frank Cain, 'MacKay, William John', *Australian Dictionary of Biography*, vol. 10, Melbourne University Press, Melbourne, 1986.

2 Bee Miles, 'I Leave in a Hurry', unpublished manuscript, Mitchell Library, ML MSS 3225, Item 1, p. 26. No record of this meeting has been identified. Over the years Bee insisted that the agreement was real and that she had regretted not asking for five years instead of three.

3 Paul Miller, 'Metamorphosis: Travel Narratives and Aboriginal and non-Aboriginal Relations in the 1930s', *Journal of Australian Studies*, no. 78, 2002, pp. 85–92.

4 Mark Finnane (ed), *Policing in Australia: Historical Perspectives*, New South Wales University Press, Sydney, 1987, p. 96; Julie Kimber, '"A Nuisance to the Community": Policing the Vagrant Woman', *Journal of Australian Studies*, vol. 34, no. 3, 2010, pp. 275–99.

5 Bernard Hesling, *The Dinkum Pommie*, Ure Smith, Sydney, 1963.

6 Stephen Garton, *Medicine and Madness*, New South Wales University Press, Sydney, 1988, p. 142.

7 Miles, 'I Leave in a Hurry', p. 4. In order to illustrate her point, Bee described a recent decision by members of 'a certain club' in Sydney, not to give lifts to women. She claimed the decision arose from a case where a woman had 'failed—failed mind you—to get a conviction against a man on the charge of assault in a car, the woman having asked for and having received a lift'.

8 Ibid., p. 21.

9 Joy Thwaite, *The Importance of Being Eve Langley*, Sydney, Angus & Robertson, 1989.

10 Miles, 'I Leave in a Hurry', p. 25.

11   Ibid., p. 60.

12   Ibid., p. 13.

13   Ibid.

14   Wendy Lowenstein, *Weevils in the Flour*, Scribe, Melbourne, 1978.

15   Kylie Tennant, *The Missing Heir*, Macmillan Australia, Sydney, 1986, pp. 80–1.

16   *Daily Standard*, Brisbane, 10 April 1934.

17   Miles, 'I Leave in a Hurry', p. 28.

18   Ibid., p. 112.

19   The Roskillys had lived in Mount Romeo since 1911. Two years after Bee's visit Lavinia Roskilly died, aged sixty-six. *Cairns Post*, 30 December 1936.

20   Ion Idriess was a hugely successful travel and adventure writer whose books continued to be popular for most of the twentieth century. Neil Jenkins knew him while he was in Cooktown writing *Men of the Jungle*. Bee thought he was a good writer but that his later works were too 'sticky'.

21   Gary Osmond, 'Bending the Ball: Racial Policy and 1930s Sport on Thursday Island', *Australian Historical Studies*, vol. 53, no. 1, 2022, pp. 5–25; Jeremy Hodes, 'Anomaly in Torres Strait: Living Under the Act and the Attraction of the Mainland', *Journal of Australian Studies*, no. 64, 2000, p. 69; Ellie Gaffney, *Somebody Now*, Aboriginal Studies Press, Canberra, 1989.

22   Miles, 'I Leave in a Hurry', p. 56.

23   Ernestine Hill, *The Great Australian Loneliness*, Robertson & Mullins Limited, Melbourne, 1948, p. 201.

24   The SDUK operated between 1826 and 1846 in Britain. Its aim was to make scientific information available through inexpensive publications for the broader population. It complemented the aims of the Mechanics Institutes.

25   Miles, 'I Leave in a Hurry', pp. 50–1.

26   Melba's family, the Dargies, had been prominent farmers in the Daly River area before settling in Darwin. Melba's sister Thelma became successful as a commercial hunter.

27   Hill, *The Great Australian Loneliness*, p. 223.

28   Miles, 'I Leave in a Hurry', p. 65.

29   R.H.B. Kearns, 'Lewis, John (1844–1923)', *Australian Dictionary of Biography*, vol. 10, Melbourne University Press, Melbourne, 1986.

30   Miles, 'I Leave in a Hurry', p. 69.

31   Tim Rowse, 'Cook, Evelyn Aufrere (Mick) (1897–1985), *Australian Dictionary of Biography*, vol. 17, Melbourne University Press, Melbourne, 2007.

32   Hill, *The Great Australian Loneliness*, p. 150.

33   Alison Holland, *Breaking the Silence: Aboriginal Defenders and the Settler State, 1905–1939*, Melbourne University Press, Melbourne, pp. 249–52.

34   Miles, 'I Leave in a Hurry', p. 84.

35   Bee Miles, 'For We Are Young and Free', Frank Johnson Papers, Mitchell Library, ML MSS 1214, Item 4.

36   Bee Miles, interview with James Ricketson, Mitchell Library, MLOH, 535/1–4.

Chapter 9: Grand Schemes

1   Kenmore Hospital, MHNSW – StAC:NRS-17418-11-447-4789.

2   Bernard Hesling, *The Dinkum Pommie*, Ure Smith, Sydney, 1963, p. 78.

3 Bee Miles, 'I Go on a Wild Goose Chase', unpublished manuscript, Mitchell Library, ML MSS 3225, Item 2, p. 4.

4 Norman Douglas (1868–1952) was a popular novelist and travel writer who lived on the island of Capri for many years. His novel *South Wind* was published in 1917 and was phenomenally successful. His private life was full of scandal with allegations of sex with under-aged minors, male and female, following him across Europe. Early in his career Jack Lindsay had been so impressed with Douglas that he dedicated one of his first novels to him. He was associated with both D.H. Lawrence and Grahame Greene. *South Wind* was one of Bee's favourite novels and she quoted it frequently.

5 John Murphy, *A Decent Provision: Australian Welfare Policy, 1870–1949*, Routledge, London, 2011, pp. 157–81.

6 Frank Huelin, *Keep Moving: An Odyssey*, Australian Book Company, Sydney p. 34.

7 Miles, 'I Go on a Wild Goose Chase', p. 18. Maurice de Abravanel was a highly acclaimed conductor who had studied under Kurt Weill. He spent two years in Australia conducting both the Melbourne and Sydney opera seasons, before joining the Metropolitan Opera in New York.

8 Jill Roe, *Stella Miles Franklin: A Biography*, Harper Collins, Sydney, 2008, p. 346.

9 Miles, 'I Go on a Wild Goose Chase', p. 27.

10 Ibid., p. 29.

11 Ibid., p. 35.

12 Ibid., p. 40.

13 Ibid., p. 41.

14 Ibid., unnumbered entry.

15 H.L. Mencken, 'The Iconoclast', *A Mencken Chrestomathy*, Alfred A. Knopf, New York, 1956, p. 17.

16 Mencken, cited in Gavin Souter, 'The Outlaw', unpublished manuscript, 1956, copy in possession of the author.

17 Bee Miles correspondence, Stephensen Papers, Mitchell Library, ML MSS 1284, Box 36.

Chapter 10: Blind Ambition

1 'Daughter Charges Assault', *Labor Daily*, 30 July 1936, p. 19.

2 'Bumper Bar Girl in Court: Bee Miles Prosecutes her Father', *Truth,* 2 August 1936, p. 4.

3 'Whistling Daughter Annoys Father', *Truth*, 19 September 1937, p. 26.

4 W.J. Miles correspondence with E. Piesse, 9 September 1936, Stephensen Papers, ML MMS 1284, Box 43.

5 Andrew Moore, *The Secret Army and the Premier*, University of New South Wales Press, Sydney, 1989, pp. 75–6.

6 Ibid., p. 161.

7 Eric Campbell, *The Rallying Point*, Melbourne University Press, Melbourne, 1965.

8 *The Bulletin*, 11 June 1925; see also J.T. Lang, *The Great Bust*, McNamara's Books, Katoomba, NSW, 1980, p. 50.

9 Craig Munro, *Wild Man of Letters: The Story of P.R. Stephensen*, Melbourne University Press, Melbourne, 1984. Information about Stephensen is largely drawn from Munro's comprehensive biography.

10   Ibid., p. 72.

11   Mikhail Bakunin (1814–1876) was a Russian revolutionary who is credited with founding the Social Anarchist Movement. A former protégé of Marx, he was expelled from the First International for his opposition to one party rule and his advocacy for a system of self-governing communes. His book *God and the State* remains in print and was a major influence on the political framework of the IWW.

12   Phillip Lindsay, *I'd Live the Same Life Over*, Hutchinson, London, 1941, p. 175.

13   Munro, *Wild Man of Letters*, pp. 138–9.

14   Egon Kisch visited Australia in 1934 as a delegate to the All Australian Congress Against War and Fascism. Before he could land, he was refused entry to Australia and famously jumped off the ship breaking his leg. He was later given a dictation test in Scottish Gaelic under the *Immigration Restriction Act* (1901) and arrested as an illegal immigrant when he refused to undergo the test. The charges were later overturned in the High Court.

15   Bee Miles correspondence with Bruce Muirden, 22 July 1965, Bruce Muirden Collection, Box 1.

16   Munro, *Wild Man of Letters*, p. 149.

17   Stephensen, *The Foundations of Culture in Australia*, W.J. Miles, Gordon, 1936, pp. 25–6.

18   W.J. Miles to Stephensen, correspondence, August 1935, Stephensen Papers, Mitchell Library, ML MSS 1284, Box 45.

19   W.J. Miles correspondence with the ANA, January 1941, Stephensen Papers, Box 41.

20   Munro, *Wild Man of Letters*, p. 173.

21   Stephensen, 'A War of Emotions', *The Publicist*, July 1939, p. 10.

22   *The Publicist*, November 1937, p. 5.

23   *Abo Call*, no. 3, June 1938, p. 2.

24   Benauster, 'Editorial', *The Publicist*, January 1938.

25   Heather Goodall, *From Invasion to Embassy: Land in Aboriginal Politics in New South Wales, 1770–1972*, Allen & Unwin, Sydney, 1996, p. 243.

26   Bain Attwood and Andrew Marcus, *The Struggle for Aboriginal Rights: A Documentary History*, Allen & Unwin, Sydney, 1999, pp. 15–17; Alison Holland, *Breaking the Silence: Aboriginal Defenders and the Settler State 1905–1939*, Melbourne University Press, Melbourne, 2019, pp. 249–52.

27   Transcript of radio interview Jack Patten and Stephensen, cited in Attwood and Marcus, *The Struggle for Aboriginal Rights*, p. 81.

28   Stephensen correspondence with Australian Aborigines League, December 1937, Stephensen Papers, Box 111.

29   Peter Lindsay, correspondence, April 1941, Stephensen Papers, Box 42. Lionel had been sending copies of *The Publicist* to Peter in London.

30   Stephensen, 'Fifty Points for Australia'.

31   Stephensen, 'A Brief Survey of Australian History', *The Publicist*, January 1938.

32   Jill Roe (ed.), *My Congenials: Miles Franklin and Friends in Letters*, Angus & Robertson, Sydney, 2010, p. 456.

33   Jack Lockyer interviewed by Craig Munro, 16 May 1977, Craig Munro Papers, Fryer Library UQFL253, Box 23, Folder 4.

34   John Benauster, 'Editorial', *The Publicist*, July 1936, p. 1.

35   Munro, *Wild Man of Letters*, p. 202.

36 The Hon. Joseph Lyons correspondence with Stephensen, 10 March 1939, Stephensen Papers, Box 42.
37 David Bird, *Nazi Dreamtime: Australian Enthusiasts for Hitler's Germany*, Australian Scholarly Publishing, Melbourne, 2012, pp. 48–9.
38 Terry Irving and Rowan Cahill, 'Welcoming the Nazi Tourist' in *Radical Sydney*, p. 223.
39 Munro, *Wild Man of Letters*, p. 204.
40 C421 item 16, NAA Canberra.
41 Ibid.
42 Bird, *Nazi Dreamtime*, p. 58.
43 C421, item 16, NAA, Canberra.

Chapter 11: Fame and Infamy

1 *Truth*, 6 March 1938.
2 P.R. Stephensen, 'Foreword', Frank Johnson Papers, Mitchell Library, MSS 1214/22, Item 2.
3 *Sydney Sun*, 16 January 1934.
4 John Kirtley was a fine book publisher who published both Jack Lindsay's and Kenneth Slessor's first books of poetry. He established Franfolico Press and, together with Jack, took the press to London in the 1920s. When he left London, his position at the press was taken over by Stephensen. Kirtley later had peripheral involvement in *The Publicist*, attended Yabber Club meetings and was close to both William and Stephensen, for whom he worked occasionally. His regular correspondence with William drew the attention of security officers and he was interned along with AFM members, although he never joined the movement. He was released after two years and the experience and the scandal left him emotionally scarred and embittered.
5 Stephensen correspondence with J. Kirtley, July 1941, Stephensen Papers, Mitchell Library, ML MSS 1284, Box 42.
6 C421, Item 40, National Archives of Australia, Canberra; David Bird, *Nazi Dreamtime: Australian Enthusiasts for Hitler's Germany*, Australian Scholarly Press, Melbourne, 2012, p. 344.
7 C421, Item 40, National Archives of Australia, Canberra.
8 C421, Item 26, National Archives of Australia, Canberra.
9 John Benauster, *The Publicist*, February 1940, p. 1.
10 C421, Item 40, National Archives of Australia, Canberra.
11 *Tweed Daily*, 19 September 1944, p. 3.
12 C421, Item 16, National Archives of Australia, Canberra.
13 Bruce Muirden, *The Puzzled Patriots*, Melbourne University Press, Melbourne, 1968, p. 4.
14 *Daily News*, 2 June 1938, p. 10.
15 *Mirror*, Perth, 28 May 1938, p. 1.
16 *Mirror*, Perth, 30 July 1938, p. 1.
17 Kenneth Slessor, 'Smith's Own Honors List', *Smith's Weekly*, 18 June 1938.
18 *The Sun*, 9 June 1939, p. 3.
19 Craig Munro, *Wild Man of Letters: The Story of P.R. Stephensen*, Melbourne University Press, Melbourne, 1984, p. 196.

20 Bede Nairn, *The Big Fella: Jack Lang and the Australian Labor Party, 1891–1949*, Melbourne University Press, Melbourne, 1986, p. 204.

21 George Mosse, *The Fascist Revolution: Towards a General Theory of Fascism*, Howard Fertig, New York, 1999, pp. 96–7.

22 Stephensen correspondence with A. Kershaw, August 1941, Stephensen Papers, Box 42.

23 William Miles correspondence with E. Piesse, October 1939, Stephensen Papers, Box 43.

24 William Miles correspondence with H. Holland, December 1941, Stephensen Papers, Box 42.

25 William Miles, Probate, NSW State Archives.

26 Marilyn Lake, 'Female Desires and the Meaning of World War II' in Joy Damousi and Marilyn Lake (eds), *Gender and War: Australians at War in the Twentieth Century*, Cambridge University Press, Melbourne, 1995, p. 68.

27 Merv Acheson, 'The Merv Acheson Story', *Jazz Magazine*, Spring, 1983.

28 Lake, 'Female Desires', p. 67.

29 Betty Roland, *The Eye of the Beholder*, Hale & Iremonger, Sydney, 1984, p. 216.

30 Stephensen, 'Fifty Points for Australia', The Publicist Publishing Co, Sydney, 1941.

31 The Australian Women's Guild of Empire was founded by Adela Pankhurst Walsh in 1928.

32 Munro, *Wild Man of Letters*, pp. 210–12.

33 Jill Roe, *Stella Miles Franklin: A Biography*, Harper Collins, Sydney, 2008.

34 C421, Item 53, National Archives of Australia, Canberra.

35 C421, Item 3, National Archives of Australia, Canberra.

36 Munro, *Wild Man of Letters*, pp. 217–18.

37 William Miles to John Kirtley, 3 June 1941, Stephensen Papers, Box 42.

38 Munro, *Wild Man of Letters*, p. 171.

39 Ibid.

40 Bruce Muirden, *The Puzzled Patriots*, p. 64.

41 Bee Miles interview with James Ricketson, 25 August 1973, Mitchell Library, MLOH, 535/1–4.

42 Jack Lockyer interviewed by Craig Munro, 16 May 1977, Sydney, Craig Munro Papers, Fryer Library, UQFL253, Box 23, Folder 4.

43 Stephensen, 'Valedictory Address', 11 January 1942, Stephensen Papers, Box 39.

44 Death of Mr W.J. Miles, *Sydney Morning Herald*, 14 January 1942; 'Woman Called a Nuisance', *Sun*, 14 January 1942.

45 Terry Irving and Rowan Cahill, 'The Battle of Bligh Street', in Terry Irving and Rowan Cahill (eds), *Radical Sydney: Places, Portraits and Unruly Episodes*, University of New South Wales Press, Sydney, 2010, p. 238.

46 *Daily Telegraph*, 20 February 1942.

47 Munro, *Wild Man of Letters*, p. 218.

48 Ibid., p. 219.

49 Ibid., p. 231.

50 C421, Item 4, National Archives of Australia, Canberra.

51 'Australia First Internees', *Smith's Weekly*, 5 September 1942.

52 Kenneth Slessor, *Of Bread and Wine: Selected Prose*, Angus & Robertson, Sydney, 1970.

53 Kenneth Slessor, 'Five Bells', in *One Hundred Poems*, Angus & Robertson, Sydney, 1944.

54 Munro, *Wild Man of Letters*, p. 240.

55 'Australia First Link—Big Money Allegation', *Sun*, 19 June 1944.

56 Munro, *Wild Man of Letters*, p. 265.

57 Ibid.

58 *Daily Telegraph*, 29 May 1965; Munro, *Wild Man of Letters*, p. 270.

59 Stephenson correspondence with B. Adamson, 30 October 1940, Stephensen Papers, Box 40.

60 Mark McKenna, *The Captive Republic: A History of Republicanism in Australia, 1788–1996*, Cambridge University Press, Melbourne, 1996, p. 217.

61 Andrew Moore, *The Secret Army and the Premier*, University of New South Wales Press, Sydney, 1989.

62 Stephensen to Jack Lindsay, cited in Munro, *Wild Man of Letters*, p. 262.

Chapter 12: A Tenant of the City

1 *Mirror*, 31 March 1945.

2 Stephen Garton, *Out of Luck: Poor Australians and Social Welfare*, Allen & Unwin, Sydney, 1990, p. 139.

3 Peter Bourke, 'The Poverty of Homelessness', in Ruth Fincher and John Nieuwenhuysen (eds), *Australian Poverty Then and Now*, Melbourne University Press, Melbourne, 1998, p. 297.

4 'Bee Decided Hospital was Home' *Sun*, 6 September 1944.

5 Carolyn Allport, 'Women and Suburban Housing: Post-war Planning in Sydney 1943–61' in Peter Williams (ed.), *Social Process and the City*, Allen & Unwin, Sydney, 1983, p. 75.

6 John Murphy, *Imagining the Fifties: Private Sentiment and Political Culture in Menzies' Australia*, University of New South Wales Press, Sydney, 2000, p. 15; Judith Brett, *Robert Menzies' Forgotten People*, Macmillan Australia, Sydney, 1992, pp. 25–7.

7 Bee Miles, 'The Cops and Me', *Weekend*, 1 December 1956, p. 7.

8 Ibid., p. 6.

9 'Kind Words', *Daily Telegraph*, 28 August 1955.

10 Bee Miles, 'Dictionary by a Bitch', unpublished manuscript, Frank Johnson Papers, Mitchell Library, ML MSS 1214/22, Item 3, p. 10.

11 Miles, 'The Cops and Me', p. 7.

12 Alma Hood, *The Bulletin*, vol. 097, no. 4950, 29 March 1975.

13 Diogenes of Sinope (circa 412–323 BC) was one of the founders of the Greek philosophical school of Cynicism. He was a controversial figure and was well known for criticising contemporary social conventions and for disrupting public lectures by distracting the audience. For a period, he lived in a pithos, a large ceramic jar, in the marketplace, to demonstrate the virtue of poverty through action.

14 'Sing When You Are Happy Cry When You Are Sad', *Daily Mirror*, 20 June 1948. In a version published eight years later, she added, 'Be discontented with what you are—morally and intellectually'.

15 George Johnston, 'Sydney Diary', *Sun*, 6 May 1948.

16 As reported in the *Canberra Times*, 12 December 1984.

17   Gavin Souter, 'Sydney is Rich in Characters', *Sydney Morning Herald*, 24 May 1958.

18   *Barrier Daily Truth*, 5 December 1944.

19   Bee Miles, 'Dictionary by a Bitch', p. 3.

20   'Bee Miles Impresses Judges', *Mirror*, 1 October 1947.

21   'Bea Miles Praised at Eisteddfod', *Sun*, 25 September 1948.

22   'Discord by Bee', *Sun*, 8 June 1947.

23   'Bee Miles fined 22 pounds', *Sun*, 18 February 1949.

24   'A Begging Charge Hurt Beatrice', *Sunday Telegraph*, 17 December 1950.

25   'Peripatetic, but No Peri', *Sun*, 3 August 1950. Bee won her appeal but was fined £1 for calling the arresting policeman 'a fool', which she admitted.

26   Gavin Souter, 'The Outlaw', unpublished manuscript, 1956, copy in possession of the author.

27   Ibid.

28   Allan Curtis, personal communication.

29   Souter, 'The Outlaw'.

30   This site is currently occupied by Woolworths.

31   Kevin Sadlier, 'Bee's Story', *Australian Magazine*, 27 April 1996.

32   Souter, 'The Outlaw'.

33   Ibid.

34   William Shakespeare, *Henry VIII*, Act 1, Scene 2.

35   Donald McLean, 'Bea Miles: The Ghost of Darlo Secondary', *Sun Herald*, 19 December 1973. Quote is from Shakespeare's *The Tempest*.

36   Bee Miles interview with James Ricketson, 25 August 1973, Mitchell Library, MLOH, 535/1–4.

37   Kevin Sadlier, 'Bee's Story'.

38   Lewis Rodd, *John Hope of Christ Church: A Sydney Church Era*, Alpha Books, Sydney, 1972.

39   John Pollard personal communication, 16 January 2022; see also John Pollard, *Exploring the Parish of Christ Church St Laurence*, St Laurence Press, Sydney, 2020.

40   Rodd, *John Hope*, p. 189.

41   John Pollard, personal communication.

42   Ibid.

43   Ibid.

44   John Lee, personal communication.

45   Rodd, *John Hope*, p. 171.

46   John Pollard, personal communication.

47   Ibid.

48   Rodd, *John Hope*, pp. 190–1.

49   Gavin Souter, *Sydney Observed*, Angus & Robertson, Sydney, 1968, p. 43.

Chapter 13: Transport Wars

1   James Homes, 'I Have Never Forgotten Bee Miles', *Canberra Times*, 1 August 1994.

2   Museums of History NSW, 'Shooting Through: Sydney by Tram', https://sydney livingmuseums.com.au/stories/shooting-through-sydney-tram

3   R. Lidden, personal communication.

4   T. Bacales, personal communication.

5   'Real Life Dramas of the Courts', *Daily Telegraph*, 12 January 1941.

6   'Tram Assault Cost Bee Five', *Truth*, 17 October 1943.

7   'Five Because She Liked Comfort', *Mirror*, 9 June 1945.

8   'Bee Miles Tired of Prison', *Sun*, 3 February 1942.

9   Jill Roe, 'Chivalry and Social Policy in the Antipodes' in Richard White and Penny Russell (eds), *Memories and Dreams: Reflections on 20th Century Australia*, Allen & Unwin, Sydney, 1997.

10 'Bee Called a Menace', *Sun*, 14 July 1946.

11 'Woman Injured in Fall from Tram', *Newcastle Morning Herald*, 27 February 1945.

12 'Bea's Bus Ride to the Police Station', *Sunday Telegraph*, 12 July 1959.

13 Robert Lidden, personal communication.

14 Stella Lees and June Senyard, *The 1950s—How Australia Became a Modern Society and Everyone Got a House and a Car*, Hyland House, Melbourne, 1987, p. 18.

15 'Bee Miles Hurt in Car Accident', *Sun*, 11 August 1947.

16 'Bea Miles Hurt', *Sydney Morning Herald*, 3 April 1950.

17 'Bea Miles Wins, Loses', *Mirror*, 12 August 1948.

18 'Sydney Diary', *Sun*, 6 May 1948.

19 'Woman Quotes Judge's Ruling on Obstruction', *Newcastle Morning Herald*, 24 December 1948.

20 'Kind Words from a Judge Stung "Bea" into Silence', *Daily Telegraph*, 28 August 1955.

21 Report of the Superintendent of Motor Transport, 1952. Parliament of New South Wales, March 1953.

22 *Daily Telegraph*, 5 June 1949.

23 'Taximan Throws Water on Woman', *Newcastle Sun*, 29 December 1950.

24 'City Notes', *Macleay Argus*, 25 February 1953.

25 'Bea Miles Hit by Cab', *Daily Telegraph*, 22 July 1955.

26 Kevin Sadlier, 'Bee's Story', *Australian Magazine*, 27 April 1996.

27 Tony Moore, *Dancing with Empty Pockets: Australia's Bohemians*, Murdoch Books, Sydney, 2012, p. 181.

28 Frank Bongiorno, *The Sex Lives of Australians*, Black Inc, Melbourne, 2012, p. 212.

29 'But "Bea" Showed She Had Lost None of Her Sting', *Daily Telegraph*, 16 October 1955.

30 *Sydney Morning Herald*, 6 October 1954.

31 Marilyn Lake, 'Female Desires: The Meaning of World War II', in Richard White and Penny Russell (eds), *Memories and Dreams: Reflections on 20th Century Australia*, p. 120.

32 *Daily Mirror*, 11 January 1956.

33 Bee Miles, 'The Cops and Me', *Weekend*, 1 December 1956, pp. 6–7.

34 'Real Life Court Dramas', *Daily Telegraph*, 22 February 1948.

35 Miles, 'The Cops and Me', p. 6.

36 Martha Rutledge, 'Meagher, James Anthony', *Australian Dictionary of Biography*, vol. 15, Melbourne University Press, Melbourne, 2000; Nancy Kessing, *Riding the Elephant*, Allen & Unwin, Sydney, 1988, pp. 63–4.

37 Michael Duffy and Nick Horden, *World War Noir: Sydney's Unpatriotic War*, New South Publishing, Sydney, 2019, p. 23.

38 John Byrell, 'Bea Miles—the Best Act in Town', *Journalist*, June/July 1987.

39   Bee Miles, 'Dictionary by a Bitch', unpublished manuscript, Frank Johnson Papers, Mitchell Library, ML MSS 1214/22, Item 3, p. 19.

40   'Called Sergeant Names', *Truth*, 12 August 1945.

41   'Bill Rodie Presents Real Life', *Daily Telegraph*, 5 June 1949.

42   'Notes from the City', 17 June 1949.

43   *Gundagai Independent*, 14 October 1946.

44   'Bill Rodie Presents Real Life', *Daily Telegraph*, 8 May 1949.

45   There are several witness accounts of Bee taking a bath and washing her clothes at Sydney Hospital, much to the annoyance of some of the doctors.

46   *Daily Mirror*, 2 October 1990.

47   'Bill Rodie Presents Real Life', *Daily Telegraph*, 16 July 1950.

48   'Peripatetic but No Peri', *Sun*, 3 August 1950.

49   *Daily Telegraph*, 22 February 1948.

50   'Asylum Won't Have Bea!', *Truth*, 14 April 1957.

51   'Bea Was Stung by a Taxi Driver', *Daily Telegraph*, 26 February 1956.

52   'Bea Miles, Now 63, Calls Off Her Private War', *Sydney Morning Herald*, 3 June 1963.

Chapter 14: Love and the Nation

1   ABC Radio interview, 1972.

2   John Ramsland, *With Just but Relentless Discipline: A Social History of Corrective Services in New South Wales*, Kangaroo Press, Sydney, 1996, pp. 157–9.

3   John Ramsland, 'Dulcie Deamer and the Women's Reformatory Long Bay', *Journal of Interdisciplinary Gender Studies*, vol. 1, no. 1, 1995, p. 37.

4   Ramsland, *With Just but Relentless Discipline*, p. 300.

5   Nerida Campbell, *Femme Fatale: The Female Criminal*, Historic Houses Trust, Sydney, 2009.

6   'Class Conscious Prisoners Out at the Bay', *Truth*, 10 August 1930.

7   Judith Allen, *Sex and Secrets: Crimes Involving Australian Women Since 1880*, Oxford University Press, Melbourne, 1990, pp. 168–80; Judith Allen, 'The Making of the Prostitute Proletariat in Early Twentieth Century New South Wales' in Kay Daniels (ed.), *So Much Hard Work: Women and Prostitution in Australian History*, Fontana Books, Sydney, 1984, pp. 192–232; Raelene Frances, *Selling Sex: A Hidden History of Prostitution*, University of New South Wales Press, Sydney, 2007.

8   Gavin Souter, 'Sydney is Rich in Characters', *Sydney Morning Herald*, 24 May 1958.

9   Bee Miles interview with James Ricketson, 25 August 1973, Mitchell Library, MLOH, 535/1–4, p. 28.

10   Bee Miles, 'The Cops and Me', *Weekend*, 1 December 1956, pp. 6–7.

11   Bee Miles, 'Dictionary by a Bitch', unpublished manuscript, Frank Johnson Papers, Mitchell Library, ML MSS 1214/22, Item 3, no page number.

12   Ramsland, *With Just but Relentless Discipline*, p. 299.

13   *Mirror*, 9 November 1958.

14   *Telegraph*, 16 October 1955.

15   Miles, 'Dictionary by a Bitch', p. 22.

16   Patrick Buckridge, 'A Bohemian Wife', *Queensland Review*, vol. 15, no. 1, 2008, pp. 51–65.

17   Miles, 'Dictionary by a Bitch', p. 12.

18 Alison Bashford and Carolyn Strange, 'Public Pedagogy: Sex Education and Mass Communication in the Mid-Twentieth Century', *Journal of the History of Sexuality*, vol. 13, no. 1, 2004, pp. 71–99.

19 Miles, 'Dictionary by a Bitch', p. 4.

20 Stephen Garton, '"Fit Only for the Scrap Heap": Rebuilding Returned Soldier Masculinity in Australia after 1945', *Gender and History*, vol. 20, no. 1, 2008, pp. 48–67; Frank Bongiorno, *The Sex Lives of Australians*, Black Inc., Melbourne, 2015, pp. 199–202.

21 Miles, 'Dictionary by a Bitch', p. 14.

22 Ibid.

23 Ibid., p. 9.

24 Ibid., p. 18.

25 Bee Miles, 'For we are Young and Free', Frank Johnson Papers, Mitchell Library, ML MSS 1214/22, Item 4.

26 Hazel Rowley, *Christina Stead*, Minerva, Melbourne, 1994, p. 474.

27 Miles, 'Dictionary by a Bitch', p. 17.

28 Philip Lindsay, *I'd Live the Same Life Over*, Hutchinson, London, 1941, p. 108.

29 Ibid., p. 103.

30 Merv Acheson, 'The Merv Acheson Story', *Jazz Magazine*, Spring 1983, p. 56.

31 Douglas Stewart, *A Man of Sydney: An Appreciation of Kenneth Slessor*, Nelson, Melbourne, 1977, p. 105.

32 Desmond Robinson, 'Happy Memories of Bee', *Sydney Morning Herald*, 7 December 1973.

33 Bee Miles correspondence with Frank Johnson, Frank Johnson Papers, Mitchell Library, ML MSS 1214/3, 4 April 1958.

34 Ibid., 13 April 1958.

35 Ibid., 30 March 1958.

36 Ibid., 18 July 1958.

37 *The Bulletin*, 8 July 1961.

38 *Sydney Morning Herald*, 12 August 1961.

39 Ibid., 5 June 1965.

40 Ibid., 30 March 1968.

41 Stephen Murray-Smith (ed.), *The Dictionary of Australian Quotations*, Heinemann, Melbourne, 1984, p. 187; Stephen Tore and Peter Kirkpatrick (eds), *The Macquarie Dictionary of Australian Quotations*, The Macquarie Library, Sydney, 1990, p. 101.

Chapter 15: To Sleep: Perchance to Dream

1 John Ramsland, *With Just but Relentless Discipline: A Social History of Corrective Services in New South Wales*, Kangaroo Press, Sydney, 1996, pp. 307–8.

2 *Truth*, 'Asylum won't have Bee', 14 April 1957.

3 Gladesville Hospital, MHNSW – StAC:NRS 5030 [3/6965] T180.

4 Ibid.

5 Ibid.

6 Paul Foley, *Encephalitis Lethargica: The Mind and Brain Virus*, Springer, New York, 2018. Information on encephalitis lethargica has been drawn largely from Dr Foley's comprehensive study along with personal communications with the author.

7   Ibid., p. 422.
8   Ibid., p. 465.
9   Gladesville Hospital, MHNSW – StAC:NRS 5030 [3/6965] T180.
10 Foley, *Encephalitis Lethargica*, p. 448.
11 Ibid., p. 499.
12 *Medical Journal of Australia* 1921, cited in ibid., p. 414.
13 Gladesville Hospital, MHNSW – StAC:NRS 5030 [3/6965] T180.
14 Ibid.
15 Ibid.
16 Stephen Garton, 'Ross, Chisholm (1857–1934)', *Australian Dictionary of Biography*, vol. 11, Melbourne University Press, Melbourne, 1988.
17 Gladesville Hospital, MHNSW – StAC:NRS 5030 [3/6965] T180.
18 Ibid.
19 *Sun*, 10 January 1932.

Chapter 16: None but Fools Would Keep

1   'Police Told "Bea" Miles Bashed', *Mirror*, 11 November 1960.
2   'The Pope? He's a Handsome Dog, Says Bee, 69', *Mirror*, 13 October 1960.
3   Kevin Sadler, 'Bee's Story', *Australian Magazine*, 27–8 April 1996.
4   Bee Miles interview with James Ricketson, 25 August 1973, Mitchell Library, MLOH, 535/1–4, p. 33.
5   *Sun Herald*, 8 December 1968.
6   'The New Bea Miles', *Sun*, 20 July 1970.
7   'The Pope? He's a Handsome Dog'.
8   *Mirror*, 22 January 1971.
9   Ian Moffitt, 'On to the Cab Rank in the Sky', undated.
10 Judy Lyons, 'How Beatrice Miles the Rebel Became a Catholic', *Catholic Weekly*, 13 December 1973, p. 13.
11 Alan Gill, 'The Church that was Home to Bea Miles', *Sydney Morning Herald*, 8 December 1957.
12 Dianne Drew, private communication.
13 Ibid.
14 Larry Writer, *Bumper: The Life and Times of Frank 'Bumper' Farrell*, Hachette, Sydney, 2011, p. 267.
15 *The Coming Out Show*, ABC, December 1975.
16 *The Bulletin*, 12 January 1974.
17 Anne Summers, 'The Other Side of History', *National Times*, 13–18 March 1978.
18 'Letters to the Editor', *Sydney Morning Herald*, 25 June 1980.
19 'Letters to the Editor' *Sydney Morning Herald*, 27 June 1980.
20 'Thumbs Down for Bea Statue', *Telegraph*, 7 December 1983.
21 Judith Allen, 'Miles, Beatrice (Bea), *Australian Dictionary of Biography*, vol. 10, Melbourne University Press, Melbourne, 1986.
22 Kate Timmins, private communication.
23 Peter Craven, 'Reading Australia—*Lillian's Story* by Kate Grenville', *Australian Book Review*, 27 May 2015.
24 'Letters to the Editor', *Sydney Morning Herald*, 21 June 1994.

25 'Letters to the Editor', *Sydney Morning Herald*, 29 June 1994.

26 Bill Barlow, 'Letters to the Editor, *Sydney Morning Herald*, 1 July 1994.

27 *Sydney Eccentrics: A Celebration of Individuals in Society*, guide, Mitchell Library.

28 Bee Miles, 'Dictionary by a Bitch', unpublished manuscript, Frank Johnson Papers, Mitchell Library, ML MSS 1214/22, Item 3, p. 11.

29 See for example Toby Creswell and Samantha Trenowith (eds), *1001 Australians You Should Know*, Pluto Press, Melbourne, 2006, p. 312. Bee is listed under the 'Crime and Law' category between Mad Dog Moran and Ivan Milat.

30 Gavin Souter, *Sydney*, Angus & Robertson, Sydney, 1965, pp. 27–8.

31 *Sydney Morning Herald*, 2 July 1994.

Index